Published by TW Publishers
E-mail: admin@publishingabook.co.za
Website: www.publishingabook.co.za
Tel: 0817319634/WhatsApp: 0782679725
Midrand, Gauteng

Lesley Meyer
Physiotherapist (special interest in chronic pain, health & wellness)
E-mail: cope.sa@vodamail.co.za
Practice number: 7237278

Disclaimer:
The purpose of this book is to educate and entertain. The author and/or publisher do not guarantee that anyone following these techniques, suggestions, tips, ideas, or strategies will become successful. The author and/or publisher shall have neither liability nor responsibility to anyone with respect to any loss or damage caused, or alleged to be caused, directly or indirectly by the information contained in this book

Also available as an e-book on Amazon Kindle & Kobo

Print ISBN: 978-0-620-75864-2/eBook ISBN: 978-0-620-75865-9

Praises for "tired of being tired to the point of being gatvol"

Lesley treated me for chronic pain in the chest area due to the broken rib and inflammation in my chest and chest muscles. After the shock of being so ill and being in constant pain I became depressed, she helped me with her "tapping" method to regain my emotional and mental health.

During that time, we discovered that I was allergic to almost everything. She assisted me in a healthy diet plan and encouraged me to stick to it, which made a huge difference in my health.

Since then she has worked with my husband, and both my daughters and the results were astonishing!!! She did not just improve our quality of life, but taught us and gave us the tools to maintain it too!!! We as a family are proof that her methods work and made a huge impact and difference in our lives. We are forever thankful that our paths crossed.

~ZELMIA BEZUIDENHOUT~

I was critically injured when I first went to see Lesley. I suffered from chronic back pain and unexplainable foot pains. Doctors believed I had arthritis and had ruined the nerves in my feet. Through her needling technique and lifestyle advice I worked my way out of my pain and into health again. Today I barely suffer from any injuries and hardly have to visit the physio (bitter-sweet). I've also gained enough strength to start participating in half marathons and high intensity training. The start of this journey would not have been possible without Lesley's continuous support and treatments.

~THANDEKA XABA~

Tired of being tired to the point of being gatvol (fed up)

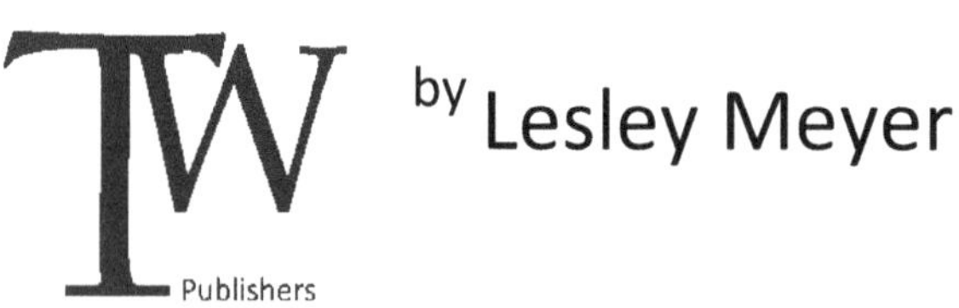

Contents

Introduction: Worth the weight in gold

Just to give you a bit of insight as to who I am and what I do, and what gives me the authority to write this book. The book which you are now holding in your hands. Is it because the title caught your eye, because you feel the same way I did?

I am a physiotherapist, but most of my patients ask me "Am I sure I am just a physiotherapist, because what I do with them is just, well, so much more?" Those are their words not mine. I always joke with them though and say, yes I am qualified as a physiotherapist, but because I have been where you are and found my way out the hole, I do a little bit more than just the physio stuff, which yes I was trained for. So my title is physiotherapist, but with a special interest in chronic pain.

I am very grateful I do what I do, as I could not imagine myself doing anything else. I absolutely love what I do and I am passionate about what I do and if I can't find what is wrong with you, I will have dreams about you and come up with all kinds of ideas that I will try out on you until we find what fits. I will relate many stories of this as you go through this book. My goal is to help my chronic pain patients who land up on my doorstep to find their way back to health and happiness. This is a long haul process and is not a quick fix. Often I will treat my patients regularly for years before we reach our final goal, but within 2-4 treatments, you can feel a difference. The main thing is that if you follow the suggestions in this book, then you will reap the benefits. It's called the slight edge. This will also be elaborated on later, as this was one of the biggest ah ha moments I had in my life.

It has been some time that I have been thinking about writing, but nothing strong enough pushed me to do so, until I was bitten by a dog and dislocated my finger. By this time I was gatvol (fed up) of being injured and having to spend years repairing what had been broken in seconds. I was just coming out of the previous slump of injury and starting to feel well enough to go for a walk and then wham, I am back on the operating table having another part fixed. So I decided that perhaps I should be sharing my story and my experiences and what I have learnt through my patients, and myself, with you.

When I say I was gatvol of being injured, it means that every 5 years I have experienced an unwanted and unexpected injury to my body and then for good measure, in-between I have experienced self-inflicted problems from things I have done that I did not think would have such dire effects. It seems I have a tattoo on my forehead that says, pick me for the disaster. The problem is that even though you are better with treatment, you are never 100% as before the injury. You retain some of the pain and deformity especially after surgery. Normal injuries you can heal 100%, a simple ankle strain, broken arm or leg that was still well aligned. The catch is to learn how to manage those problems where permanent deformation or pains are a result of the injury.

I am currently treating a patient who suffers from severe debilitating headaches that cause dizziness and tinnitus (ringing in the ears). He responded very quickly to treatment, because I was able to identify and teach him where his pain was coming from. Once he knew where it was coming from, I then showed him what to do when he felt his headache start. Now he says instead of his headaches taking away his life, when he feels the pain he pinches the muscle and within 5 minutes his headache is gone. We have also changed his diet and provided specific supplements for him and he said that he has not felt this good in a very long time. His problems and pains were so bad that he was medically boarded from work. Hopefully with him continuing to release the muscle that is causing all the problems and continuing with his diet and supplementation, he should have a great retirement, where pain will no longer rule his life. He will feel like a king and in control of what is happening in his body as he knows what to do to fix the problem instantly.

I always say to my patients. "If you know where the pain is coming from and what caused it, you are half way there. Because, when you know where it is coming from, I can show you what to do to fix it. The other 50% is just doing what I advise you to do and voila, problem solved."

It has been almost a year since my dog bite injury, and this specific injury led me to write this book as this was the final straw. I have suffered from chronic pain since 1995 after a major car accident. It took 10 years before I found relief from my pain. I tried many different ways to relieve the pain and many different specialists and Doctors and alternative therapies and home remedies, until I found what worked for me. What I learnt was that each item does work, but you need to find which one you gel with, that you will be prepared to try and then do it until you are better. Sometimes no one thing will work, but a combination of different things. It is not necessarily just a physical problem or an emotional problem, but a combination of everything, which together gives you the overall picture of what you feel.

So each time I went to a specialist or Doctor, or physio, I listened to what they said. Some of it I felt was true and others I felt was not true. We know when the problem started and what the cause of the problem was. Sometimes when you don't know what the cause was, if you are guided through the time frame with some specific questions, it will dawn on you and one can pinpoint exactly what it was. I had a lady who came to me many years ago with a hip pain, but she said that she did not know why it was sore. When I started asking her specific questions like, have you had this pain before, or when did this pain start for the first time, she suddenly remembered she had had a stiff hip 3 months prior, after walking on the beach. The beach was steep and she had walked with the one leg shorter than the other for more than a kilometre. She had really enjoyed the walk and had not felt any pain until the next day when the hip that was higher was stiff. After a few days this pain went away and she didn't think of it again. This is enough to cause havoc in your hip. So a few sessions of dry needling and massage and her hip was jumping for joy again.

Another patient was complaining of neck pain and did not know the cause. It was a new pain and had only been there for 2 days, so I asked her what she had done two days prior to it being sore. Here she mentioned that she had been carrying around a camera for two days taking photos, the camera had been slung over just the one shoulder, the one that was now giving her neck pain. Most problems sneak up on you like this. Usually two days prior to the pain starting think of the activity that caused the pain. So a small car accident and two days later you are stiff, or a fall and two days later you are stiff, or spring cleaning and two days later..... Get the idea?

In my case I knew my problems were from my car accident. I had broken my ribs and the muscles on my back had gone into such spasm that they had formed tight bands. Many of the physiotherapists said that these tight bands were fibrous and there was nothing more that they could do for me. They obviously have not experienced pain that drives you mad and makes you cry because nothing you are doing is working. This type of pain is just unbearable. But thank goodness 10 years after my accident, I found a physio who had specialized in IMS (intramuscular stimulation) and he needled my entire body in 45 min, and for the first time in a long time I was pain free. But this was just the start. If you do not respond to treatment, it is due to a metabolic insufficiency, meaning that your vitamins and minerals in your body are lacking or are excessive. This can be rectified with diet and supplementation. So I went on courses through the Check institute where I learnt about nutrition and lifestyle coaching.

Chronic pain is not just a physical entity, as long duration pain becomes a mental and emotional problem as well. If you are going through a lot of stress, be it work stress, relationship stress, burglary or breakup, these emotional situations that you go through can cause a simple injury which takes place at the same time, to become a chronic physical problem. Many patients I have worked with, and once again their stories will come to light later in the book, who have not responded to normal treatment have all been cases where they have experienced emotional trauma during the physical injury. Once I realized that the person is a physical, mental, emotional being with chemicals galore, I went on a hunt to learn the technique called EFT, (Emotional freedom technique), NLC (Nutrition and lifestyle coaching), IMS (intramuscular stimulation), and courses on supplementation and health.

As if the car accident in 1995 was not enough, I seem to attract some or other injury or system error every 5 years, to a point where I have permanent damage and am out of action for at least 2 weeks. It has been so bad that last year I went through an emotional time out session where I spent 6 months analysing my life with the help of an EFT practitioner to guide me through my thought processes. I can really recommend having outside help, be it a psychologist, or EFT practitioner, when you are running your thoughts through your head on a stuck program, it is really useful having outside input to change the way you perceive the situation. I am currently reading a book titled *"Living on purpose through pathological positivity." by Paul H Jenkins*. What he says in the book really made me think. He mentioned that we all have things we go through, but it is our choice how we respond to the situation.

The car accident that I had, could have been viewed as the worst thing that ever happened to me, as I have had substantial continuous pain since, that stopped me from doing any sport I was passionate about. I could have chosen to be miserable about the pain and crawl into bed and bemoan the fact that I have pain and become very depressed and horrible to be around. However, I saw my accident as the best thing that happened to me (pathological positivity). Mad perhaps, but because I am in the medical field and I am a physio, it led me down a path of self-exploration of how far I can push myself before I get the dreaded pain, and if I get the dreaded pain, what to do to fix it. Many people have not experienced what I have and thus do not know what the patients are complaining about when they mention the dead arms, or the pins and needles or the pain that feels like your arm is falling off, or the pain that feels like your coccyx is breaking or someone is stabbing you in the chest, or your legs are giving you the creeps because they are irritating the living daylights out of you. I have had them all and some.

This pain has led me to help my patients on a deeper level, because when they come in and describe their pain, I can definitely add to it and describe it in more detail, where they are nodding their head along with me, going, how did you know? Well I got the T-shirt and have worn it through already.

If you choose to be negative about your situation, it will make your healing impossible. You need to find some silver lining in the situation you find yourself in. It may even be that you have learnt what pain is and can be empathetic towards others in pain. It may be that you overcome your pain and are able to help someone else get over theirs. It may be that you learn that you are unhappy in your marriage or work and that is what is causing your pain. So you have two choices, either change your job or get a divorce, or if that is not an option, then you need to change the way you see your work or marriage. Get help and change the way you think about things, because you can only heal yourself when you are able to change the thoughts that created the problem in the first place.

There was another book I read that said, don't wait for others to change the things you are complaining about. The author was talking about how people have a tendency to say work is so boring, it would be much better if they had pizza on Fridays, or had team building events, etc. Another example would be how you perhaps complain about the litter around your work building or in your suburb. Don't just sit back and expect someone else to fix the problem, you must become part of the solution.

I was sitting on the beach when I was reading this book. I was disgusted by the amount of litter that was lying around on the beach and we had to look for a clear spot to sit. When I read this part of the book, I realized that I was sitting there complaining about the fact that the beach was dirty and expecting someone else to fix the problem. I know there are workers who collect the litter, but I do not think there are any that collect litter on this specific beach, and they are not always available. So I mentioned to my son, that perhaps we should think about doing something about the beach ourselves. I said that I didn't want to make it my new job, as I was there to have holiday, but if I took two plastic bags every day and filled them up with rubbish, while we were walking along the beach admiring the shells, then that would be good enough. While we walked along the beach, we picked up our two bags of rubbish over a course of 10 days. We had people stop us regularly asking us what we were doing. They were so impressed that we even had a little girl join us the one day to pick up her two bags of rubbish. By the end of the 10 days holiday, our section of the beach was rather tidy and it was far more comfortable to sit on the clean beach.

This is not where it stopped. When I returned home and mentioned it to a few of my patients, I got told stories of what they had seen and what they were going to do to do their bit. The one patient told me of a gentleman who cycled to work every day. He would cycle through a forest area that was filled with rubbish. He decided that every day he would take two packets to fill, and then continue on his route. One day a motorist stopped to ask him what he was doing, after the explanation this motorist took it upon himself to add his two packets to the equation and within a few months the forest was beautifully clean and the birds started to return to nest.

I also told this story to a priest who then took it upon herself to organize once a month a clean-up session of a specific area. But this did not stop there. She arranged that some members of the congregation would drive around collecting the beggars off the street and get them to come and help pick up rubbish. After a few hours of rubbish collection, they would then arrange that the beggars would be given a nice meal. Thus we get the beggars feeling as if they have something to offer and then rewarding them for their effort.

She is also working with other dynamic people in her church to create cleanliness in Olivenhoutbosch, which has a huge refuse problem. They have a school they started there and are planning on having a shop on the school premises. This shop will be stocked through donations from the congregation and anyone else who would like to make a donation of food, clothing, toys, and other items. The shop will be divided into three isles, a red isle, blue isle and a yellow isle. The children then require monopoly type money (Pendulas), red, blue and yellow coloured money, to be able to shop in this shop. To get these Pendulas, they need to bring in clean recyclable rubbish. This rubbish is weighed and Pendulas are given to them according to the weight brought in. If you have yellow money you can buy products from the yellow isles and blue, from blue isle and red from red isle. The yellow represents that you buy for your own family, the blue represents that you buy for someone else and the red represents that you can buy something for yourself. I am really impressed with this whole concept and three of these shops are being opened in 2016 and their aim is to open another three every year. I can only foresee how the townships can become beautiful clean areas and people may start to show initiative in keeping the community clean, but also in thinking of others and not just of themselves all the time.

These books have really helped in the way I think about life in general. It took me 6 months to analyse my life. I was seriously wondering what I was doing for fun, as it felt as if I was in the proverbial rat race. I seemed to have lost the plot. It felt as if I had no joy in my life and everything that I did enjoy before was just draining me of energy and was no fun anyway, so why bother doing them. It was also during this time that my mom approached me to take over her physio practice. She is reaching retirement age and works full time in the children's ward, treating chests. The problem was that if I took over this practice, I would only be able to do my work that I love to do, in the summer months and in the winter I would have to dedicate myself to only do the hospital work. It is guaranteed work, but if there is no one to do the work, then I would have to work, that means I would have to work every public holiday, including Christmas and new year and Easter. I would have to be on standby 365 days of the year and if a locum was unable to work because she was sick or such, I would have to drop everything I was doing and go and treat the kids at the hospital.

This was a very heavy burden. Take a job that is lucrative and guaranteed work and payment, but involves 365 days commitment and it is not something I am passionate about, and you never know what your day is going to look like. Or continue with what I am doing, which is my passion and has a set time period, so my diary is planned every day? I was running these through my head constantly, as I almost felt that I needed to be doing both, but knew it was not possible, but didn't want to give up my own work to do this, but felt that I needed to because of the money. Very confusing!

It was during this time that I was reading yet another book. And this is the most mind blowing information I got out of the book, which helped me make the decision that I am going to be doing for the rest of my career. It was a quadrant. At the top quadrant was LIKE TO, LOVE TO and at the bottom quadrant was HATE TO, HAVE TO. In each quadrant you need to write all the things in your life that you like to do or love to do and again at the bottom of the quadrant hate to and have to. What I realized was that I hated doing the hospital work. It was the unplanned diary and never knowing how many kids were going to be there for the day. It was the stress of not knowing if I would finish in time to fetch the kids from school. I do not feel it is right that they must sit around not knowing when I will be there. If I have said I will be there at 13h30, then that is the time I must arrive not later.

Also I am not passionate about treating chests, as I always get sick and one has difficult parents on occasion. I knew that if I continued to treat the kids in the ward, I would become miserable, as I would have to give up what I enjoy and love and like to do, to do something I hate and would have to do. jOnce I had done this exercise, I knew that there was no way that I would do the children's ward, and I was able to tell my mother that she would need to find an alternative person to take over form her as I would not even want to run it.

So what do I mean that I suffer every 5 years with some or other injury? Well it all started in 1995 with the car accident. Prior to that

I had broken my arms 6 times (not through child abuse), just pure fall and break my arm scenario. I was a walking Kiewiet (lapwing bird/walking skinny person). I had had encephalitis when I was three, and a knee injury from a hockey ball during an intense game, and a few migraines from Grade 7 – 11, but other than that, I was rather healthy. Then I had my car accident.

Chapter 1
The start of your journey

As I am writing this chapter I am feeling really good. My life is great and I am having fun, enjoying my work and looking forward to this year ahead to learn everything I have lined up to learn and experience and do. I am a bubbly person and enjoy lifting other peoples' spirits and moods. Of course this has to be done with a lot of talking and explaining and the conversations I have with my patients are often deep and meaningful, but we are always able to bring the silver lining into any negative situation and look at it differently so that they are able to recover from their difficult life experiences just as I have.

Even when I have been through so many different traumas, they have not been able to break my spirit and if I have been a bit low, it was never long enough to become a permanent fixture. But just long enough to teach me an invaluable lesson and enable me to use this information for teaching and educating and helping anyone who is prepared to listen to me babble away bits of madness amongst deep truths.

It was during one of my self-inflicted traumas that my spirit was momentarily broken for a few years, but I see it as a propportunity to enable me to empathize with my patients, as I know exactly how they are feeling and thinking. Each trauma I have been through I have managed to change it into a propportunity and this is not a spelling mistake! A propportunity is a problem that has been changed into an opportunity. Frankly I like this new word.

I am sure many of you are tired, and sore and feel you have lost yourself somewhere along the way. You have forgotten who you are. All you know is that you are not yourself and you are tired of feeling this way. You are irritated with yourself, you constantly accuse yourself of being lazy and no good, because you are not doing the normal number of activities that you would usually do in the past. Basically you are tired of being tired to the point of being gatvol (fed up).

I have just recovered from feeling like this and would like to help you do the same. When I was this tired I was so cross with myself, because I had been trying to accomplish something that was just not happening, which was totally unknown to me. I felt like a naffy dog barking around and everyone just wanting to kick me in the teeth to shut up. I would get frustrated and cry from anger at myself, but I could not do anything about it, because I felt confused and totally exhausted.

It went on for about 2 years before I decided that there must be something physically wrong with me, but there was nothing concrete, it was just a bunch of little irritating things that weren't going right, things that one would not normally go to the doctor for. Apart from the fatigue I had chronic sinus and little small dry itchy patches on my skin, almost like little eczema spots. I had restless legs and struggled to sleep at night, lying awake for hours before falling asleep and then waking at 3 in the morning and waiting for the alarm to go off to get going for the day. I would find any opportunity to lie down, to try and sleep but could not sleep, and exercise was a curse word. I tried walking around the block, but this made it worse and I would find any excuse to simply sit still.

When I went to the Doctor he did some blood tests and found that I had adrenal fatigue. What was interesting was when he was asking me about my time line. Take a moment to think and reflect on, what incident caused your fatigue or medical problem. Most of you have already figured it out, but there are some that have not even thought to do this.

A time line is basically your life on a straight line. So you analyse your life from before you were born till where you are now. When I talk about before you were born, it means, what were your parents health like, did they have any medical problems that were there when they decided to have a baby. Were they depressed, did they want you, what was the pregnancy like. This could influence your body in that you may have deficiencies already. There are literature studies that state if you have adrenal fatigue and become pregnant, your baby can have adrenal insufficiency and will suffer from low cortisol levels which can compromise the ability to handle stress. The child could be more susceptible to becoming ill from stress.

You will gain the most benefit from this book if you can pinpoint the origin of your problem. If you know what the problem is, then you are 50% of the way to resolving it.

In this time line, you need to jot down any event that may have happened to you at the top of the line, then under the line, you right down any symptoms that you suffer from and when they started. If you can't think of events that may have happened but remember that you were depressed in Std. 7 or started with bowel problems when you were 8, then you have the symptom at a certain age, and need to then think about what was happening in your life during that time period. Perhaps you were in a stressful home environment. Perhaps you were constantly moving and felt insecure. Maybe you were a sickly child or a teacher said something to you that stuck in your head and became a belief you have. It can be a number of different things that may have occurred and one needs to determine what they are so that thinking and emotional patterns around past situations can be adjusted.

I have added my time line for you to see what I mean. I also find it much easier to do something when you already have an idea of what is expected of you.

Incident	Year/age	Complaint/problems
Encephalitis	3yrs old	Global trophoedema
Broke R arm	6Yrs	
Broke R arm	7yrs	
Broke R arm	8yrs	
Broke both arms	9 yrs.	
Broke R arm	Std. 3	
German measles	Std. 4	Migraines started (till std. 8)
	Std. 6	Menstrual cycle started
Hockey ball Knee injury	Std. 11	Knee pain & swelling & weakness
Car accident	Second yr	broken ribs, Headaches, body pains, knee pain, face injury, Broken finger
Over worked, dirty environment	1998	Sinus infection/Antibiotics, constipation
Went overseas 8months		weight gain, sinus infection
1st kidney stone, studied further	2000	
2nd Kidney stone,	2001	Swelling in legs more pronounced
Moved to UK for 4 yrs		weight gain, swelling of eyes, sinus, diarrhea, heart palpitations, body cramping, increased global pains, P&N arms and legs
bicycle accident	2004	Whiplash injury, dizziness, headaches, stomach cramping, other pains increased
Travel to NY	2005	Severe swelling of legs
returned to SA, pregnancy	2006	back pain, body pain, headaches
	2007	Incontinence from tear during birth, 2 years
3rd & 4Th kidney stone, death of cat/uncle/aunt	2010	
started dancing & Harvested Eggs	2012	Fatigue, more body pain, swelling of legs,
Harvested twice	2013	weight gain, migraines, menstrual
Loss of triplets	2014	problems, hot flushes, mood swings, aggression, irritation, intolerance to noise (radio)
Dog bite dislocation	2015	Finger stiffness and loss of function Fatigue continued, peri-menopause, Osteopenia, gall stones
Injury of lumbar/sacral area gardening	2016	Dead feet, coccyx pain, sore quads

The second thing that I want you to do is complete the HAQ assessment form. You know where you have come from and what has happened to you to cause all the problems. This graph will now show you how bad things are. It is an objective means of measuring if you are improving. So great to do every 6 months when you have been implementing the healing strategies. It will categorize your body into low, medium and high priority and obviously the higher the priority the worse your condition. So be as honest with yourself as you can when answering these questions.

It is said that the body has the ability to heal itself if given the opportunity to do so; however you can't change if you have the same mind-set in which you created the problem. So by doing your time line, you are giving your body the opportunity to find the cause of the problem and then this book can give you the tool in which to change the mind-set and belief and this results in your body healing. It is the most amazing and wonderful thing to see happen and it does not take long to change a mind-set when using the EFT tool and getting some insight into your past. I have seen it countless times in my patients and am amazed each time.

People will ask you if you have changed your hair or done something different, because you look different. Your whole facial expression changes and you feel lighter and happier and you feel like the old happy you, a much better you.

I am pleased that you are taking the time to do your time line, and HAQ, it was a huge eye opener for me and although it has taken me 4 years to recover once I was diagnosed and there are still some obstacles I need to overcome, it has been well worth the journey both physically and emotionally. I have really come to understand who I am and what my purpose here on earth is, and this is part of my purpose, to help as many people as I can to find themselves and to heal from within. This is a never ending journey as you are constantly learning and doing and wanting to do more, but you cannot do anything if you do not have the health to do it, no matter how much you want it to happen.

Good luck on your journey, it is going to be the best one ever.

Health Appraisal Questionnaire

Name ______________________________ Date ______________

DIRECTIONS

This questionnaire asks you to assess how you have been feeling during **the last four months**. This information will help you keep track of how your physical, mental and emotional states respond to changes you make in your eating habits, priorities, supplement program, social and family life, level of physical activity and time spent on personal growth. All information is held in strict confidence. Take all the time you need to complete this questionnaire.

For each question, circle the number that best describes your symptoms:

0 = No or Rarely – You have never experienced the symptom or the symptom is familiar to you but you perceive it as insignificant (monthly or less)

1 = Occasionally – Symptom comes and goes and is linked in your mind to stress, diet, fatigue or some identifiable trigget

4 = Often – Symptom occurs 2-3 times per week and/or with a frequency that bothers you enough that you would like to do something about it

8 = Frequently – Symptom occurs 4 or more times per week and/or you are aware of the symptom every day or it occurs with regularity on a monthly or cyclical basis

Some questions require a YES or NO response: 0 = NO 8 = YES

PART 1

SECTION A

	No/Rarely	Occasionally	Often	Frequently
1. Indigestion, food repeats on you after you eat	0	1	4	8
2. Excessive burping, belching and/or bloating following meals	0	1	4	8
3. Stomach spasms and cramping during or after eating	0	1	4	8
4. A sensation that food just sits in your stomach creating uncomfortable fullness, pressure and bloating during or after a meal	0	1	4	8
5. Bad taste in your mouth	0	1	4	8
6. Small amounts of food fill you up immediately	0	1	4	8
7. Skip meals or eat erratically because you have no appetite	0	1	4	8
Total points				

SECTION B

	No/Rarely	Occasionally	Often	Frequently
1. Strong emotions, or the thought or smell of food aggravates your stomach or makes it hurt	0	1	4	8
2. Feel hungry an hour or two after eating a good-sized meal	0	1	4	8
3. Stomach pain, burning and/or aching over a period of 1-4 hours after eating	0	1	4	8
4. Stomach pain, burning and/or aching relieved by eating food, drinking carbonated beverages, cream or milk, or taking antacids	0	1	4	8
5. Burning sensation in the lower part of your chest, especially when lying down or bending forward	0	1	4	8
6. Digestive problems that subside with rest and relaxation	(0)No			(8)Yes
7. Eating spicy and fatty (fried) foods, chocolate, coffee, alcohol, citrus or hot peppers causes your stomach to burn or ache	0	1	4	8
8. Feel a sense of nausea when you eat	0	1	4	8
9. Difficulty or pain when swallowing food or beverage	0	1	4	8
Total points				

SECTION C

	No/Rarely	Occasionally	Often	Frequently
1. When massaging under your rib cage *on your left side*, there is pain, tenderness or soreness	0	1	4	8
2. Indigestion, fullness or tension in your abdomen is delayed, occurring 2-4 hours after eating a meal	0	1	4	8
3. Lower abdominal discomfort is relieved with the passage of gas or with a bowel movement	0	1	4	8
4. Specific foods/beverages aggravate indigestion	0	1	4	8
5. The consistency or form of your stool changes (e.g., from narrow to loose) within the course of a day	0	1	4	8

SECTION C (cont.)

	No/Rarely	Occasionally	Often	Frequently
6. Stool odor is embarrassing	0	1	4	8
7. Undigested food in your stool	0	1	4	8
8. Three or more large bowel movements daily	0	1	4	8
9. Diarrhea (frequent loose, watery stool)	0	1	4	8
10. Bowel movement shortly after eating (within 1 hour)	0	1	4	8
Total points				

SECTION D

	No/Rarely	Occasionally	Often	Frequently
1. Discomfort, pain or cramps in your colon (lower abdominal area)	0	1	4	8
2. Emotional stress and/or eating raw fruits and vegetables causes abdominal bloating, pain, cramps or gas	0	1	4	8
3. Generally constipated (or straining during bowel movements)	0	1	4	8
4. Stool is small, hard and dry	0	1	4	8
5. Pass mucus in your stool	0	1	4	8
6. Alternate between constipation and diarrhea	0	1	4	8
7. Rectal pain, itching or cramping	0	1	4	8
8. No urge to have a bowel movement	(0)No			(8)Yes
9. An almost continual need to have a bowel movement	(0)No			(8)Yes
Total points				

PART II

	No/Rarely	Occasionally	Often	Frequently
1. When massaging under your rib cage *on your right side*, there is pain, tenderness or soreness	0	1	4	8
2. Abdominal pain worsens with deep breathing	0	1	4	8
3. Pain at night that may move to your back or right shoulder	0	1	4	8
4. Bitter fluid repeats after eating	0	1	4	8
5. Feel abdominal discomfort or nausea when eating rich, fatty or fried foods	0	1	4	8
6. Throbbing temples and/or dull pain in forehead associated with overeating	0	1	4	8
7. Unexplained itchy skin that's worse at night	0	1	4	8
8. Stool color alternates from clay colored to normal brown	0	1	4	8
9. General feeling of poor health	0	1	4	8

PART II

	No/Rarely	Occasionally	Often	Frequently
10. Aching muscles not due to exercise	0	1	4	8
11. Retain fluid and feel swollen around the abdominal area	0	1	4	8
12. Reddened skin, especially palms	0	1	4	8
13. Very strong body odor	0	1	4	8
14. Are you embarrassed by your breath?	0	1	4	8
15. Bruise easily	(0)No			(8)Yes
16. Yellowish cast to eyes	(0)No			(8)Yes

Total points

PART III

SECTION A

	No/Rarely	Occasionally	Often	Frequently
1. Feel cold or chilled – hands, feet or all over – for no Apparent reason	0	1	4	8
2. Your upper eyelids look swollen	0	1	4	8
3. Muscles are weak, cramp and/or tremble	0	1	4	8
4. Are you forgetful?	0	1	4	8
5. Do you feel like your heart beats slowly?	0	1	4	8
6. Reaction time seems slowed down	0	1	4	8
7. In general, are you disinterested in sex because your desire is low?	0	1	4	8
8. Feel slow-moving, sluggish	0	1	4	8
9. Constipation	0	1	4	8
10. Dryness, discoloration of skin and/or hair	(0)No			(8)Yes
11. Have you noticed recently that your voice is deepening?	(0)No			(8)Yes
12. Thick, brittle nails	(0)No			(8)Yes
13. Weight gain for no apparent reason	(0)No			(8)Yes
14. Outer third of your eyebrow is thinning or disappearing	(0)No			(8)Yes
15. Swelling of the neck	(0)No			(8)Yes

Total points

SECTION B

	No/Rarely	Occasionally	Often	Frequently
1. Lingering mild fatigue after exertion or stress	0	1	4	8
2. Do you find that you get tired and exhaust easily?	0	1	4	8
3. Craving for salty foods	0	1	4	8
4. Sensitive to minor changes in weather and surroundings	0	1	4	8
5. Dizzy when rising or standing up from a kneeling position	0	1	4	8
6. Dark bluish or black circles under your eyes	0	1	4	8
7. Have bouts of nausea with or without vomiting	0	1	4	8
8. Catch colds or infections easily	(0)No			(8)Yes
9. Wounds heal slowly	(0)No			(8)Yes
10. Your body or parts of your body feel tender, sore, sensitive to the touch, hot and/or painful	0	1	4	8
11. Feel puffy and swollen all over your body	0	1	4	8
12. Skin is gradually tanning without exposure to sun or the ingestion of high levels of carotene-rich foods (e.g., daily carrot juice intake) or supplements	(0)No			(8)Yes

Total points

PART IV

SECTION A

When you miss meals or go without food for extended periods of time, do you experience any of the following symptoms?

	No/Rarely	Occasionally	Often	Frequently
1. A sense of weakness	0	1	4	8
2. A sudden sense of anxiety when you get hungry	0	1	4	8
3. Tingling sensation in your hands	0	1	4	8
4. A sensation of your heart beating too quickly or forcefully	0	1	4	8
5. Shaky, jittery, hands trembling	0	1	4	8
6. Sudden profuse sweating and/or your skin feels clammy	0	1	4	8
7. Nightmares possibly associated with going to bed on an empty stomach	0	1	4	8
8. Wake up at night feeling restless	0	1	4	8
9. Agitation, easily upset, nervous	0	1	4	8
10. Poor memory, forgetful	0	1	4	8
11. Confused or disoriented	0	1	4	8
12. Dizzy, faint	0	1	4	8
13. Cold or numb	0	1	4	8
14. Mild headaches or head pounding	0	1	4	8
15. Blurred vision or double vision	0	1	4	8
16. Feel clumsy and uncoordinated	0	1	4	8

Total points

SECTION B

	No/Rarely	Occasionally	Often	Frequently
1. Frequent urination during the day and night	0	1	4	8
2. Unusual thirst—feeling like you can't drink	0	1	4	8
3. Unusual hunger—eating all the time	0	1	4	8
4. Vision blurs	0	1	4	8
5. Feel itchy all over	0	1	4	8
6. Tingling or numbness in your feet	0	1	4	8
7. Sense of drowsiness, lethargy during the day not associated with missing meals or not sleeping	0	1	4	8
8. Eating starchy foods, even if they are healthy and unprocessed (like rice, corn, beans, whole wheat or oats), causes you to gain weight or prevents you from losing weight	(0)No			(8)Yes
9. Sores heal slowly	(0)No			(8)Yes
10. Loss of hair on your legs	(0)No			(8)Yes

Total points

PART V

SECTION A

	No/Rarely	Occasionally	Often	Frequently
1. Feel jittery	0	1	4	8
2. First effort of the day causes pain, pressure, tightness or heaviness around the chest	0	1	4	8
3. Exhaustion with minor exertion	0	1	4	8
4. Heavy sweating (no exertion, no hot flashes)	0	1	4	8
5. Difficulty catching breath, especially during exercise	0	1	4	8
6. Heart pounding, sensation of heart beating too quickly, too slowly or irregularly	0	1	4	8
7. Swelling in feet, ankles and/or legs comes and goes for no apparent reason	0	1	4	8

Total points

PART V (cont.)

SECTION B

	No/Rarely	Occasionally	Often	Frequently
1. Muscle pain at rest	0	1	4	8
2. Cramp-like pains in your ankles, calves or legs	0	1	4	8
3. Numbness, tingling and prickling sensation in hands and feet	0	1	4	8
4. Cold feet and/or toes appear blue	0	1	4	8
5. Brief moments of hearing loss	0	1	4	8
6. Nausea comes and goes quickly (unrelated to eating)	0	1	4	8
7. Feel worse standing: legs get heavy and fatigued	0	1	4	8
8. Leg discomfort or fatigue relieved by elevating legs	0	1	4	8
9. Fingers and toes get numb in cold weather even when protected	0	1	4	8
10. Notice changes in your ability to feel pain or differentiate between sensations of hot or cold	(0)No			(8)Yes
11. Body hair (on arms, hands, fingers, legs and toes) is thinning or has disappeared	(0)No			(8)Yes
12. Do you notice a decline in your ability to make decisions, concentrate, focus attention or follow directions?	(0)No			(8)Yes

Total points

SECTION B (cont.)

	No/Rarely	Occasionally	Often	Frequently
12. Do you become suddenly scared for no reason?	0	1	4	8
13. Do you break out in a cold sweat?	0	1	4	8
14. "Butterflies in your stomach," nausea and/or diarrhea	0	1	4	8

Total points

SECTION C

	No/Rarely	Occasionally	Often	Frequently
1. Do you feel pent up and ready to explode?	0	1	4	8
2. Are you prone to noisy and emotional outbursts?	0	1	4	8
3. Do you do things on impulse?	0	1	4	8
4. Are you easily upset or irritated?	0	1	4	8
5. Do you go to pieces if you don't control yourself?	0	1	4	8
6. Do little annoyances get on your nerves and make you angry?	0	1	4	8
7. Does it make you angry to have anyone tell you what to do?	0	1	4	8
8. Do you flare up in anger if you can't have what you want right away?	0	1	4	8

Total points

PART VI

SECTION A

	No/Rarely	Occasionally	Often	Frequently
1. Family, friends, work, hobbies or activities you hold dear are no longer of interest	0	1	4	8
2. Do you cry?	0	1	4	8
3. Does life look entirely hopeless?	0	1	4	8
4. Would you describe yourself as feeling miserable and sad, unhappy or blue?	0	1	4	8
5. Do you find it hard to make the best of difficult situations?	0	1	4	8
6. Sleep problems—too much or too little sleep	0	1	4	8
7. Changes in your appetite and weight	(0)No			(8)Yes
8. Lately you've noticed an inability to think clearly or concentrate	(0)No			(8)Yes
9. Difficulty making decisions and/or clarifying and achieving your goals	(0)No			(8)Yes

Total points

SECTION B

	No/Rarely	Occasionally	Often	Frequently
1. Does worrying get you down?	0	1	4	8
2. Does every little thing get on your nerves and wear you out?	0	1	4	8
3. Would you consider yourself a nervous person?	0	1	4	8
4. Do you feel easily agitated?	0	1	4	8
5. Do you shake and tremble?	0	1	4	8
6. Are you keyed up and jittery?	0	1	4	8
7. Do you tremble or feel weak when someone shouts at you?	0	1	4	8
8. Do you become scared at sudden movements or noises at night?	0	1	4	8
9. Do you find yourself sighing a lot?	0	1	4	8
10. Are you awakened out of your sleep by frightening dreams?	0	1	4	8
11. Do frightening thoughts keep coming back in your mind?	0	1	4	8

PART VII

	No/Rarely	Occasionally	Often	Frequently
1. Eyes water or tear	0	1	4	8
2. Mucus discharge from the eyes	0	1	4	8
3. Ears ache, itch, feel congested or sore	0	1	4	8
4. Discharge from ears	0	1	4	8
5. Is your nose continually congested?	0	1	4	8
6. Are you prone to loud snoring?	(0)No			(8)Yes
7. Does your nose run?	0	1	4	8
8. Nosebleeds	(0)No			(8)Yes
9. Hoarse voice	0	1	4	8
10. Do you have to clear your throat?	0	1	4	8
11. Do you feel a choking lump in your throat?	0	1	4	8
12. Do you suffer from severe colds?	(0)No			(8)Yes
13. Do frequent colds keep you miserable all winter?	(0)No			(8)Yes
14. Flu symptoms last longer than 5 days	(0)No			(8)Yes
15. Do infections settle in your lungs?	(0)No			(8)Yes
16. Chest discomfort or pain	0	1	4	8
17. Do you experience sudden breathing difficulties?	0	1	4	8
18. Do you struggle with shortness of breath?	0	1	4	8
19. Difficulty exhaling (breathing out)	0	1	4	8
20. Breathlessness followed by coughing during exertion, no matter how slight	0	1	4	8
21. Inability to breathe comfortably while lying down	0	1	4	8
22. Do you cough up lots of phlegm?	0	1	4	8
23. Can you hear noisy rattling sounds when breathing in and out?	0	1	4	8
24. Are you troubled with coughing?	0	1	4	8
25. Do you wheeze?	0	1	4	8
26. Do you have severe soaking sweats at night?	0	1	4	8
27. Do your lips and/or nails have a bluish hue?	0	1	4	8
28. Are you sleepy during the day?	0	1	4	8

PART VII (cont.)

	No/Rarely	Occasionally	Often	Frequently
29. Do you have difficulty concentrating?	0	1	4	8
30. Eyes, ears, nose, throat and lung symptoms seem associated with specific foods like dairy or wheat products	(0)No		(8)Yes	
31. Eyes, ears, nose, throat and lung symptoms are associated with seasonal changes	(0)No		(8)Yes	

Total points

PART VIII

1. Involuntary loss of urine when you cough, lift something or strain during an activity	0	1	4	8
2. Mild lower back ache or pain	0	1	4	8
3. Abdominal achiness or pain	0	1	4	8
4. Pain or burning when urinating	0	1	4	8
5. Rarely feel the urge to urinate	0	1	4	8
6. Feel the need to urinate less than every two hours during the day or night	0	1	4	8
7. Strong smelling urine	0	1	4	8
8. Back or leg pains are associated with dripping after urination	0	1	4	8
9. Sore or painful genitals	0	1	4	8
10. Urine is a rose color	0	1	4	8
11. Sudden urge to void causes involuntary loss of urine	0	1	4	8
12. Generalized sense of water retention throughout your body	0	1	4	8

Total points

PART IX

SECTION A

1. Bones throughout your entire body ache, feel tender or sore	0	1	4	8
2. Localized bone pain	0	1	4	8
3. Hands, feet or throat get tight, spasm or feel numb	0	1	4	8
4. Difficulty sitting straight	0	1	4	8
5. Upper back pain	0	1	4	8
6. Lower back pain	0	1	4	8
7. Pain when sitting down or walking	0	1	4	8
8. Find yourself limping or favoring one leg	0	1	4	8
9. Shins hurt during or after exercise	0	1	4	8

Total points

SECTION B

1. Are you stiff in the morning when you wake up?	0	1	4	8
2. Difficulty bending down and picking up clothing or anything from the floor	0	1	4	8
3. Joint swelling, pain or stiffness involving one or more areas (fingers, hands, wrists, elbows, shoulders, toes, arches, feet, ankles, knees or ankles)	0	1	4	8
4. Joints hurt when moving or when carrying weight	0	1	4	8
5. A routine exercise program, like daily walking, causes your knees to swell or hurt	0	1	4	8
6. Difficulty opening jars that were previously easy to open	0	1	4	8
7. Discomfort, numbness, prickling or tingling sensation, or pain in neck, shoulder or arm	0	1	4	8

SECTION B (cont.)

	No/Rarely	Occasionally	Often	Frequently
8. Intermittent pain or ache on one side of head spreading to cheek, temple, lower jaw, ear, neck and shoulder	0	1	4	8
9. Difficulty chewing food or opening mouth	0	1	4	8
10. Difficulty standing up from a sitting position	0	1	4	8
11. Shooting, aching, tingling pain down the back of leg	0	1	4	8
12. Is it difficult to reach up and get a 5-pound object like a bag of flour from just above your head?	(0)No		(8)Yes	
13. Injure, strain or sprain easily	(0)No		(8)Yes	

Total points

SECTION C

1. Muscles stiff, sore, tense and/or achy	0	1	4	8
2. Burning, throbbing, shooting or stabbing muscle pain	0	1	4	8
3. Muscle cramps or spasms (involuntary or after exertion/exercise)	0	1	4	8
4. Is muscle pain or stiffness greater in the morning than other times of the day?	0	1	4	8
5. Specific points on body feel sore when pressed	0	1	4	8
6. Feel unrefreshed upon awakening	0	1	4	8
7. Headaches	0	1	4	8
8. Pain at the sides of your head or in your face especially when awakening	0	1	4	8
9. Your jaw clicks or pops	0	1	4	8
10. Muscle twitch or tremor (eyelids, thumb, calf muscle)	0	1	4	8
11. Irresistible urge to move legs	0	1	4	8
12. Legs move during sleep	0	1	4	8
13. Unpleasant crawling sensation inside calves when lying down	0	1	4	8
14. Hand and wrist numbness or pain (e.g., interferes with writing or with buttoning or unbuttoning your clothes)	0	1	4	8
15. Feeling of "pins and needles" in your thumb and first three fingers	0	1	4	8
16. Pain in forearm and sometimes in shoulder	0	1	4	8

Total points

PART X

SECTION A

1. Head feels heavy	0	1	4	8
2. Dizziness	0	1	4	8
3. Difficulty bending over, standing up from sitting, rolling over in bed and/or turning your head from side to side	0	1	4	8
4. Your hands tremble, ever so slightly, for no apparent reason	0	1	4	8
5. You feel like you're wearing heavy weights on your feet when walking	0	1	4	8
6. Bump into things, trip, stumble and feel clumsy	0	1	4	8
7. Difficulty breathing	0	1	4	8
8. Difficulty swallowing	0	1	4	8
9. People tell you to speak up because they have trouble hearing you	0	1	4	8
10. Speaking and forming words does not feel automatic	0	1	4	8
11. Need 10-12 hours of sleep to feel rested	0	1	4	8

PART X (cont.)

SECTION A (cont.)

	No/Rarely	Occasionally	Often	Frequently
12. Lack strength (your grip is weak, holding your head or picking your arms up takes effort)	0	1	4	8
13. Hands get tired when you write and your handwriting is less legible and smaller than it used to be	(0)No			(8)Yes
14. Muscles in arms and legs seem softer and smaller	(0)No			(8)Yes
15. Is your eyesight, sense of smell and taste or ability to hear not as sharp as it used to be?	(0)No			(8)Yes
16. Do you find yourself moving slower than you used to?	(0)No			(8)Yes

Total points

SECTION B

	No/Rarely	Occasionally	Often	Frequently
1. Difficulty absorbing new information	0	1	4	8
2. Tend to forget things	0	1	4	8
3. Trouble thinking or concentrating	0	1	4	8
4. Easily distracted	0	1	4	8
5. Do you have a tendency to become frustrated quickly?	0	1	4	8
6. Inability to sit still for any length of time, even at mealtime	0	1	4	8
7. Finishing tasks is easier said than done	0	1	4	8
8. Do you have more trouble solving problems or managing your time than usual?	0	1	4	8
9. Low tolerance for stress and otherwise ordinary problems	0	1	4	8

Total points

PART XI

Men Only

	No/Rarely	Occasionally	Often	Frequently
1. Sensation of not emptying your bladder completely	0	1	4	8
2. Need to urinate less than 2 hours after you have finished urinating	0	1	4	8
3. Find yourself needing to stop and start again several times while urinating	0	1	4	8
4. Find it difficult to postpone urination	0	1	4	8
5. Have a weak urinary stream	0	1	4	8
6. Need to push or strain to begin urinating	0	1	4	8
7. Dripping after urination	0	1	4	8
8. Urge to urinate several times a night	0	1	4	8

Total points

PART XII

Women Only

(Menopausal women should skip to Sections E and F)

SECTION A

Do you persistently experience any of these symptoms within three days to two weeks *prior to menstruation?*

	No/Rarely	Occasionally	Often	Frequently
[A]				
1. Anxious, irritable or restless	(0)No			(8)Yes
2. Numbness, tingling in hands and feet	(0)No			(8)Yes
3. Easy to anger, resentful	(0)No			(8)Yes
4. Aggressive or hostile toward family/friends	(0)No			(8)Yes
[B]				
5. Abdominal bloating, feeling swollen (e.g., feet)	(0)No			(8)Yes
6. Temporary weight gain	(0)No			(8)Yes
7. Breast tenderness, swelling	(0)No			(8)Yes
8. Appearance of breast lumps	(0)No			(8)Yes
9. Discharge from nipples	(0)No			(8)Yes
10. Nausea and/or vomiting	(0)No			(8)Yes
11. Diarrhea or constipation	(0)No			(8)Yes
12. Aches and pains (back, joints, etc.)	(0)No			(8)Yes
[C]				
13. Craving for sweets	(0)No			(8)Yes
14. Increased appetite or binge eating	(0)No			(8)Yes
15. Headaches	(0)No			(8)Yes
16. Being easily overwhelmed, shaky or clumsy	(0)No			(8)Yes
17. Heart pounding	(0)No			(8)Yes
18. Dizziness or fainting	(0)No			(8)Yes
[D]				
19. Confused and forgetful to the point that work suffers	(0)No			(8)Yes
20. Overwhelmed with feelings of sadness and worthlessness	(0)No			(8)Yes
21. Difficulty sleeping or falling asleep	(0)No			(8)Yes
22. Engaging in self-destructive behavior	(0)No			(8)Yes

Total points

SECTION B

Do you experience any of these symptoms *during your period?*

	No/Rarely	Occasionally	Often	Frequently
1. Cramping in lower abdomen or pelvic area	(0)No			(8)Yes
2. Lower abdominal pain is sharp and/or dull or intermittent	(0)No			(8)Yes
3. Bloating and sense of abdominal fullness	(0)No			(8)Yes
4. Diarrhea or constipation	(0)No			(8)Yes
5. Nausea and/or vomiting	(0)No			(8)Yes
6. Low back and/or legs ache	(0)No			(8)Yes
7. Headaches	(0)No			(8)Yes
8. Unusual fatigue (take naps) resulting in missed work	(0)No			(8)Yes
9. Painful and/or swollen breasts	(0)No			(8)Yes
10. Scanty blood flow	(0)No			(8)Yes

Total points

SECTION C

	No/Rarely	Occasionally	Often	Frequently
1. Painful or difficult sexual intercourse	0	1	4	8
2. Low abdominal, back and vaginal pain throughout the month	0	1	4	8
3. Pelvic pressure or pain while sitting down or standing up, relieved by lying down	0	1	4	8
4. Vaginal bleeding other than during your period	0	1	4	8
5. Painful bowel movements	0	1	4	8
6. Difficult (straining) urination	0	1	4	8
7. Abnormal vaginal discharge	0	1	4	8
8. Offensive vaginal discharge	0	1	4	8
9. Vaginal itching or burning with or without intercourse	0	1	4	8
10. Pain during periods is getting progressively worse	(0)No			(8)Yes
11. Profuse or prolonged menstrual bleeding	(0)No			(8)Yes
12. Unable to get pregnant	(0)No			(8)Yes

Total points

PART XII (cont.)

SECTION D

	No/Rarely	Occasionally	Often	Frequently
1. Absence of periods for six months or longer	(0)No		(8)Yes	
2. Periods occur irregularly (e.g., 3 to 6 times a year)	(0)No		(8)Yes	
3. Profuse heavy bleeding during periods	0	1	4	8
4. Menstrual blood contains clots and tissue	0	1	4	8
5. Bleeding between periods can occur anytime	0	1	4	8
6. Periods occur greater than every 35 days	(0)No		(8)Yes	
7. Intense upper stomach pain, lasting several hours at the time you ovulate (approximately day 14 of your cycle)	0	1	4	8
8. Bleeding occurs at ovulation (approximately day 14 of your cycle)	0	1	4	8
9. Monthly abdominal pain without bleeding	0	1	4	8
10. Abundant cervical mucus	0	1	4	8
11. Acne and/or oily skin	0	1	4	8
12. Overwhelming urges for sexual intercourse	0	1	4	8
13. Aggressive feelings	0	1	4	8
14. Increased growth of dark facial and/or body hair	(0)No		(8)Yes	
15. Poor sense of smell	(0)No		(8)Yes	
16. Voice is becoming deeper	(0)No		(8)Yes	
17. Breasts seem to be getting smaller	(0)No		(8)Yes	
18. Receding hairline	(0)No		(8)Yes	

Total points

SECTION E

	No/Rarely	Occasionally	Often	Frequently
1. Vaginal discharge	0	1	4	8
2. Vaginal secretions are watery and thin	0	1	4	8
3. Vaginal dryness	0	1	4	8
4. Sexual intercourse is uncomfortable	0	1	4	8

SECTION E (cont.)

	No/Rarely	Occasionally	Often	Frequently
5. Interest in having sex is low	0	1	4	8
6. Engorged breasts	0	1	4	8
7. Breast tenderness, soreness	0	1	4	8
8. Difficulty with orgasm	0	1	4	8
9. Vaginal bleeding after sexual intercourse	0	1	4	8
10. Do you skip periods?	(0)No		(8)Yes	
11. The length (number of days) of your period varies month to month, with the number of days of bleeding getting fewer	(0)No		(8)Yes	

Total points

SECTION F

	No/Rarely	Occasionally	Often	Frequently
1. Sense of well-being fluctuates throughout the day for no apparent reason	0	1	4	8
2. Sudden hot flashes	0	1	4	8
3. Spontaneous sweating	0	1	4	8
4. Chills	0	1	4	8
5. Cold hands and feet	0	1	4	8
6. Heart beats rapidly or feels like it is fluttering	0	1	4	8
7. Numbness, tingling or prickling sensations	0	1	4	8
8. Dizziness	0	1	4	8
9. Mental fogginess, forgetful or distracted	0	1	4	8
10. Inability to concentrate	0	1	4	8
11. Depression, anxiety, nervousness and/or irritability	0	1	4	8
12. Difficulty sleeping	0	1	4	8
13. Conscious of new feelings of anger and frustration	0	1	4	8
14. Skin, hair, vagina and/or eyes feel dry	0	1	4	8
15. Stopped menstruating around six months ago, yet still experience some vaginal bleeding	(0)No		(8)Yes	

Total points

Please mark an "X" to indicate areas where you feel pain, swelling or discomfort, or areas of your skin that have changed color or texture (e.g., moles, rashes, etc.). Describe what you feel or observe in your own words. Write anywhere in this area.

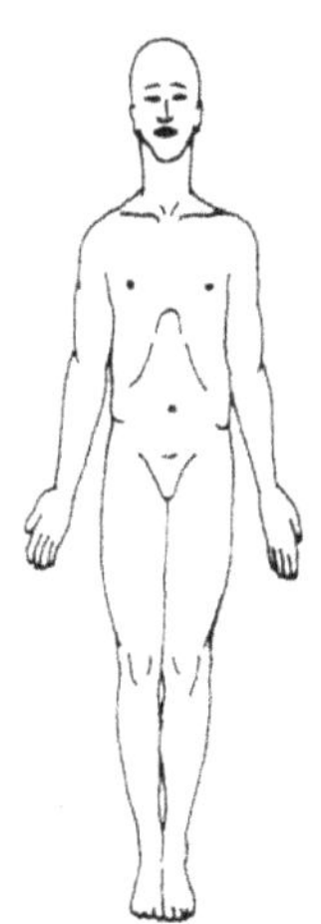

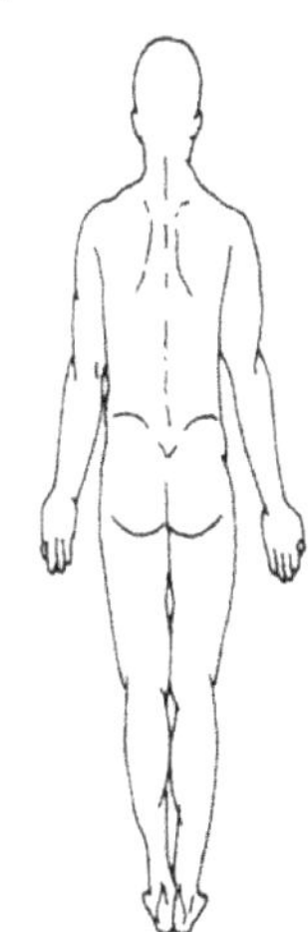

RETEST DATE ____/____/____

INITIAL TEST DATE ____/____/____

NAME ____________________

Health Appraisal Graph

Section	Category													Initial Test Score	Retest Score
XII Female	F. Estrogen/ Progesterone Decline	120	96	72	48	24	20	16	12	8	6	4	2		
	E. Ovarian Function	88	74	60	46	32	26	20	14	8	6	4	2		
	D. Hormone Balance	144	116	88	60	32	26	20	14	8	6	4	2		
	C. Reproductive Tissue Inflammation	76	60	44	28	12	10	8	6	4	3	2	1		
	B. Menstruation	80	64	48	32	16				8					
	A. Premenstrual Balance	176	142	108	74	40	32	24	16	8					
XI Male	Prostate Health	64	50	36	22	8	7	6	5	4	3	2	1		
X CNS & Brain	B. Cognition	72	62	52	42	32	28	24	20	16	12	8	4		
	A. Central Nervous System	128	100	72	44	16	14	12	10	8	6	4	2		
IX Musculoskeletal	C. Muscle & Nerves	112	88	64	40	16	14	12	10	8	6	4	2		
	B. Connective Tissue	104	80	56	32	8	7	6	5	4	3	2	1		
	A. Bone Integrity	72	56	40	24	8	7	6	5	4	3	2	1		
VIII Uro-logical	Kidney & Bladder	96	80	64	48	32	26	20	14	8	6	4	2		
VII Immune	Eyes, Ears, Nose, Throat & Lungs	248	200	160	120	100	80	60	30	15	10	8	2		
VI Mood	C. Anger	64	51	38	25	12	11	10	9	8	6	4	2		
	B. Anxiety	112	89	65	43	20	18	16	14	12	9	6	3		
	A. Depression	72	59	46	33	20	18	16	14	12	9	6	3		
V Cardio-vascular	B. Circulation	96	72	48	24	16	14	12	10	8	6	4	2		
	A. Heart	56	45	34	23	12	11	10	9	8	6	4	2		
IV Glucose Regulation	B. Dysglycemia–E	80	66	52	38	24	22	20	18	16	12	8	4		
	A. Dysglycemia–L	128	102	76	50	24	22	20	18	16	12	8	4		
III Endocrine	B. Adrenal	96	72	48	24	16	14	12	10	8	6	4	2		
	A. Thyroid	120	98	76	54	32	28	24	20	16	12	8	4		
II Liver/ GB	Hepatobiliary Function	120	94	68	42	16	14	12	10	8	6	4	2		
I Gastrointestinal (GI)	D. Colon	72	58	44	30	16	14	12	10	8	6	4	2		
	C. Small Intestine & Pancreas	80	64	48	32	16	14	12	10	8	6	4	2		
	B. GI Inflammation	72	56	40	24	8	7	6	5	4	3	2	1		
	A. Gastric Function	56	44	32	20	8	7	6	5	4	3	2	1		

0

HIGH PRIORITY **MODERATE PRIORITY** **LOW PRIORITY**

Initial Test Score Retest Score

Chapter 2
Start of my journey

It was March here in South Africa and I was rushing home to the farm, and driving along the dirt road a tad on the fast side. The grass in March is very high, so high that you do not see any traffic on the side of the road or traffic heading into the main road. Suddenly out of no-where a little boy (10yrs) turned into the main dirt road on a quad bike. I was right on top of him. I had to suddenly swerve out to avoid hitting him and slammed on my breaks, which caused the breaks to lock and send me out of control into a skid. I hit the gravel embankment made from the scraped gravel on the side of the road, which launched my car into the air. The car hit the ground and because it was a little Beatle VW with that round roof, it rolled several times before it came to a standstill in the veld on its wheels.

I am sure the little boy got the fright of his life as he rushed home to fetch his dad. In the mean time I was analysing the damage. I was in my second year of physiotherapy and had recently been taught what happens in the emergency room with people who come in after an accident. So I took a look at my right ring finger. Yes definitely broken, looks rather ugly and out of position. Knee bleeding, not sure how bad that is, but feels not too bad. Mind you nothing felt that bad, as my adrenaline had kicked into overdrive. A wonderful mechanism in the body; I then lifted my shirt to discover a black swelling over my entire rib area on the right. Oh dear, that does not look good. By this time the little boy's dad had arrived and was trying to make small talk about the old hockey stick that had been flying around the back of the car.

How I manage to stay calm and not freak out in situations like these are beyond me, as I have seen many people who become hysterical and cry or scream. The only time I became hysterical was when I broke my arm in Std. 3 as it was rather odd shaped. It looked like it had two elbows, which freaked me out, which made me scream hysterically to a point where my dad had to give me a slap to come to. Here I was calm and was wondering how things happened so fast but yet so slow. It was like I saw the whole accident happen in slow motion, but it was over in seconds. I am astounded at how quickly it takes to get hurt, but how long it takes to get better.

While I was sitting in the bug, the stranger was trying to take my pulse with his thumb, so I informed him that you can't feel a pulse with your thumb as you already have your own pulse in your thumb and to use his index finger. I don't remember anything else, and did not see or hear the helicopter land. I do not know how long it took to arrive, and don't really remember anything else the man was saying as I am sure I blacked out. I must have briefly woken up as I remember the hunky paramedic who had saved my life. It must have been when he put a needle in my chest to get equilibrium back in my lungs as the one had collapsed. I did not even notice this, but was told after. This was done as I had a pneumothorax on the right and my mediastinum had shifted which is very dangerous.

In normal language this means my lung had collapsed on the right due to the broken ribs which caused the blood to fill my lung cavity. This caused my wind pipe to shift to the side of my throat, blocking the air entry. If you do not correct the pressure in the chest, by putting a needle in the chest, you die. This happens quite quickly, so I think that helicopter got there just in time.

Apparently my dad drove past when all this was taking place, I never noticed as I was unconscious again. He came running through the veld with his bare feet. (Our South Africans in Pretoria are famous for going bare feet to where ever you want to go. It's not a poor thing; it is just a cultural thing. We have tough feet because of it and we like to go bare foot. It is a topic we often joke about with visitors from different countries or even visitors from the Cape.)

As he was not allowed to come with in the helicopter, he charged after the helicopter to follow me to the hospital. My dad is a great doctor too and he has the memory of an elephant and phenomenal general knowledge. I am sure he has some sort of photographic memory. I remember my brother asking him what a really difficult word meant. My dad rattled off the meaning, to which my brother said, not possible and hauled out the dictionary. Much to his disgrace, my dad had described the word verbatim out the dictionary, my dad just laughed at this.

We are always phoning my dad for his opinion on any medically related injury, or problem. We have this theory in our house that each of us has a purpose to help the others. I have a very big family, two brothers and two sisters and little old me stuck in the middle of the bunch of them. We had a third little brother, but he drowned when he was one and I was seven. My oldest sister is a chemical engineer and has to give advice on finances and shares, she's good with money. My other sister is a vet; she gives advice on our sick animals. My younger brother is the one that gets blamed for anything that goes wrong, from who ate the chocolate to who broke the light. But he is also good at helping us with computer related problems or cell phones or other electronic items around the house. And my little brother, he is the whit of the family, always coming up with funny comments. I think he is the cleverest of the bunch of us as he always knew all the answers to the show,

"Who wants to be a millionaire". He also completed the exam for "Mensa", the clever people club, just to see if he was clever enough to do it. Once he passed he was quite happy to just be.

Personality wise, I would say he is definitely a phlegmatic, my eldest sister is a melancholy/choleric, my other sister is a choleric/choleric, my brother is a choleric/melancholy and my dad is a choleric and my mother a melancholy and I am a sanguine/melancholy.

Phlegmatic are people who don't like to upset the apple cart, they are quite easy going and don't mind doing whatever is on the go, or sometimes just prefer to stay home doing nothing. One must not underestimate them though as if they feel strongly enough about something, they will go out of their way to get the task done. If however they do not see why they should do the task then they will never get round to doing it.

Choleric is a person who is very strong willed and they are never wrong. It is always their way or the high way. They come across as being very aggressive and people are scared to approach them. You never want to be on the bad side of a choleric person.

Melancholy is a person who is very organized; their desk is efficiently neat and organized. They know exactly who said what when and they never forget what they have done, because they have always written a report about it and filed it away in the perfect location. They like to keep stats and have their life planned out very well for the next 10 years, and have already made contingency plans for when something goes wrong because they have foreseen every possible problem. They do not like change. They also tend to be a little more on the pessimistic side of things.

Sanguine is the belle of the ball. They are the ones that never stop talking. They can never find their keys or anything else on a daily basis. They even forget where they have parked their car and may not know what car they drive, other than the blue one or the red one. They make lots of promises in good faith but then forget they made the promise and sometimes don't pull through. They are the people who lift any environment and people are attracted to their happy bubbly personalities as they make great friends, because they never keep a grudge because they don't remember who did what to them.

I may not have a large general knowledge outside my field of expertise, but hey that doesn't really matter when you can help people get better and you are the belle of the ball. I remember my brother saying to my mother the one day after I had helped him through a difficult situation using EFT. "Lesley may be weird, but she is actually quite clever". Hee hee, this was truly wonderful to hear from my brother.

Back to my accident, sad to say I don't really remember the helicopter ride, what a pity as I hear it cost a fortune, thank goodness for medical aid. But when I arrived at the emergency part of the hospital there were doctors everywhere. They were prodding me and asking me where the pain was to determine how bad the damage was, I was agreeing with their format of evaluation. We had literally been taught the week before what the Doctors would do in this situation. So the Doctor would squeeze my legs and ask, is there any pain here? NO. Then he would squeeze my thighs, any pain here? No. Then he would push my pelvic bones towards each other, any pain here? No. This all means that my legs and my pelvis were fine, no broken bones here. Press the abdomen, is there any pain here? No, thus no internal damage of my organs, this is very important.

Writing about my accident in this book made me reflect and ponder a lot on my own medical problems that I have discovered over the years and some of them could definitely be linked to the car accident. The shaking and tumbling of the car could have caused my left ovary to get stuck behind my uterus. This was only picked up when I harvested my eggs 17 years later, but it makes a lot of sense. It's the only injury that was rough enough to shake all my organs around inside and put them in new places. My kidneys also got shaken into distraction.

As he was prodding the bottom half of my body, under my watchful agreement and practical hands on learning, another doctor was checking out my ribs on the right. He needed to put in an underwater drain, Ooh, that's interesting. I am not sure if he gave me local anaesthetic before cutting a hole between my 5th and 6th rib, but I felt no pain. He then inserted a pipe connected to a bottle and voila the blood started draining out my chest. Wow, that's interesting. It was super cool watching how they were fixing me up. I am sure a lot of you are going, gross; I would faint if I saw blood. This sounds so gory, but hey, that's why I am in the medical profession and not you. I even got a thermal blanket, which I am sad to say I never got to see as it never came with me when I was transferred to the normal ward.

After many X-rays and endless doctors ensuring I had no other broken bones, I was wheeled up to ICU. Here I was watched with a beady eye for about three days. I don't really remember much of it. I think I must have been sleeping for most of the time.

I also remember having severe right shoulder pain. The poor shoulder must have taken a hammering against the door, so I begged the sisters to get me a hot water bottle. There is nothing more soothing than a hot pack on sore muscles. They had to improvise and heated up a bag of saline, which worked like magic. My diagnosis was that I had 6 broken ribs, but they were broken in the front and the back, so in effect 12 broken ribs. A bashed up face that was very swollen with a very red eye, a broken right ring finger and broken wrist and a cut open knee. I was battered and bruised and it was going to take a long time to recover from this injury. Broken ribs are the most painful thing I have experienced, and the pain lasts very long and the recovery is slow and difficult with added complications that never receded.

After the three days in ICU, they moved me down to the normal ward. Here I had to get my first shower after the accident. I was very glad of this as I still had sand in my hair from the roll in the veld. But after such a big accident, you have to be with someone when you get up for the first time, and there is no way that you can bath or wash yourself. The reason for the extra person, is that when you stand up for the first time, you usually faint, with the change in blood pressure, and that would be very painful and could cause a lot more damage. My hand was bandaged, my knee was bandaged and I was useless. It was refreshing to have that shower and I do remember feeling light headed with the heat of the water and I was able to sit on a stool in the shower with the bandages all held out the way of the water.

One of the days I remember lying in the bed, but I had slid down the bed and couldn't push myself up to get more comfortable. I was sore and I couldn't reach the call button, so I was lying there sobbing with the pain, when a nurse walked by and helped me up in the bed. She was muttering about the fact that she thought I had been spoilt in ICU with the one on one attention and that I was in the normal ward now and I must get on with my life and not be so dependent on other people.

You are not there because you are well, you are there because you are very sick and you need to be dependent on them to help you get better. She obviously has not been in a car accident and felt that excruciating pain, nothing compares to that pain, not even child birth. Not kidney stones, not a broken arm, nothing. The pain from breaking my ribs was painful with every breath I took and was painful with the smallest movement I made. Don't even talk about the coughing; you try your utmost not to cough. I was crying because it was so sore and I could not help myself into a more comfortable position. I could not push on my broken hand as it was too painful and swollen. I could not kick with my leg as it was too painful. I could not sit upright using my stomach as my ribs were too painful. I could not roll on my side as my ribs were too painful.

I do not think I had that ICU withdrawal symptom as it had only been 3 days that I was in ICU and not months. Frankly, you would cry too if you could not move and you were too sore to push the pain button or reach the call button and you could not even call out because it would be too sore to shout loudly because of the ribs, if you were wondering why I didn't call out. I was even trying my best not to cry, because even that was too painful to do.

What I was grateful for during that painful experience in the hospital, was the soft sheep skin under my buttocks which my mom had specially brought for me. Within three days of only lying on my back, I had already started developing sores on my bony sacrum. The start of a bed sore if not treated properly. One would think you only got those in old people. Sad to say, anyone can get bed sores if they do not move position regularly. They are quite a serious complication of not being able to move. Hence why we have nursing staff to help turn patients who are unable to turn themselves, or rub ointment on the patients' backs when they bath them, or have the Physios come and do passive movements and get people out of the bed while they are in hospital. All a necessary evil!

I also remember the physio that came. She made me sit over the edge of the bed and percussed me on my back with saline steaming up my nose. Although it was literally only 5 minutes, I hated it, as I am sure all of you hate it when we come to your bedsides. It was darn sore, each thud of her palm on my back reverberating through my ribs, and afterwards there was no way that I could suppress the cough that came up to excrete the phlegm. She had shown me to grab a pillow to push against my ribs to hold them tight before I coughed. There is no time to grab anything when the cough just comes. So I would learn to just grab my ribs with my hands as I coughed. That was the best compromise I could come up with, but it seemed to be effective enough. I later mastered the art of using the whole side of my arm to support the ribs over a larger area.

It was not long before I went home; I think I was a total of 5 days in the hospital. I was at home for about 4 weeks before going back to university. Luckily 2 weeks of that was holidays, so I didn't miss too much work and when I got back I had oral exams to catch up with everyone. The examiner asked me what one does in the emergency room after an accident, so I scored 100% there.

At this stage of the game, we had not learnt yet how long it takes for bones to grow back together. Since then my knowledge has expanded. I have learnt you have 4 weeks attachment and 6 weeks consolidation for the upper limbs and 6 weeks attachment and 12 weeks consolidation for the lower limbs. That is if you have normal Vit D levels. So at 4 weeks after my accident I decided that I was ready to play a hockey game.

No one had told me that I couldn't. So if you do your math here, my finger would have just attached itself and was still too unstable and my ribs were just as shocking. So I felt my ribs burning like mad during the game and after the game noticed that my finger didn't look right. It had made a funny dent, but it was not sore, so I didn't ask anyone about it and just carried on. Lack of patient compliance is one of the most prominent causes of failure in treatments and procedures.

When I went for my check-up the doctor informed me that they had to re-break my finger as it had set wrong. Hence the funny look. So 5 months after my accident I had to have my finger re-broken and reset and then I followed the rules to the T. My ribs at this stage had overlapped and were also growing on skew, probably also from the hockey game, but who knows. Unfortunately nothing can be done about that, I did try. I asked thoracic surgeons their opinion, and they all said, "Sure we just remove the rib." Now this is not an answer for me, because if you remove the rib you will change your rib structure and your chest will fall in on itself. So your back will develop a severe scoliosis.

That can only cause more pain. My idea was to break my ribs again, and pull them apart for the one centimetre and then put wire around it to hold it in place. Apparently this could not be done as the clips or wires could move into the lungs.

Since my ribs grew on overlapping each other, it means that my ribs were pulling my spine out of alignment and I now have a 16 degree scoliosis in my thoracic region and a corrective curve in my lower thoracic lumbar junction area of 12 degrees. This means I have an S shaped spine. Because of this, my muscles on the right side of my spine next to my shoulder blade would go into severe spasms, especially if the weather was cold or if I was sitting in a funny position. As I know how to manage it, I no longer have that severe pain, but still get discomfort from time to time.

Because of the nature of my injuries, about a year down the line I developed severe headaches. These would be elicited from any form of sport, so if I played hockey, that night I would be out of action with a severe headache. If I walked for 10-15 minutes on uneven surfaces outside, I would have a headache. If I sat too long to study, I would have a headache. It was horrendous. It would wake me from my sleep, I would have to take 2 Tenstons and sit up watching TV with a hot pack on my head and wait for the headache to go, then I could go back to sleep. This would take between two hours to 6 hours.

My pains gradually got worse, not only would I get headaches, but if I sat for too long my buttocks would go dead and even my legs. When I worked, I would feel the nerves in my arms pulling and it was very uncomfortable. If I lay on my sides my arms would go dead and my ribs would click. When I sat watching TV my legs would feel irritated and I would have to kick them out and fidget with the legs, restless legs. When it was cold, my back would cramp and I was in a lot of pain.

I still tried to play hockey as it was my passion. I remember the one game my calves, hamstrings and quads all cramping at the same time, this was horrible. It was so bad that I told the goalie that I would cover the box as I could hardly run anymore. The next day I could hardly walk as my legs were not just stiff sore they were just plain horrible sore. I was unable to climb up or down stairs as I had such severe pain in my ITB at the side of my knees and my calves were excruciatingly sore.

I was due to work the weekend and our hockey game was the Thursday night before. So Saturday morning I went to work and remember driving from hospital to hospital. I started early in the morning and every stop I made took me about 5 minutes to get out the car as it was so painful. I wanted to cry through each treatment I gave, as my muscles were so sore that I did not know what to do. I only finished at 6pm and by the time I got home I was crying from the pain. It was one of my worst days ever. It almost felt as if I had severe flu, the pain was so intense.

It was round about this time that I started looking for Physios to treat me. I went to all the Physios I knew and they used to say to me that I had fibrosis of the muscle on my back. This was over the area that my back would cramp. There was nothing that they could do for the fibrosis and that I must learn to live with the pain. I tell you no sane person can live with that kind of pain. It is not possible. As the pain was triggered by any sport or any activity, I stopped doing all forms of sport. It was not worth the pain. I had at this stage learnt about Dry needling and was begging the Physios to needle the area, but none of them liked needles and always told me that they would like to try other things first. Well, during the treatment, it felt great, but by the time I got back home, my pain was the same as before I went for treatment. I would then try another physio, the one would do Cranio-sacral, the other would do Pilates, but nothing got rid of my pain. These are all valuable techniques and are very effective, but they were not effective for me, so I continued with my search.

I went to Chinese doctors and drank funny smelly concoctions that made the entire house stink and made me vomit, hence that didn't last long and didn't help. I went to a chiropractor that injected me with funny stuff in my spine, which made me no better and I am convinced that it elicited my kidney stones. I went to massage therapists and they stretched me so badly into pain that I had severe pain for a month. Every time I changed my work area, as I was a locum. I would try the Physios there, hoping someone would do the needles on me.

I then went to the UK and worked there for 4 years and this is where I met the genius Prof Chan Gunn. I decided to try the physio who had been lecturing on the course and after 6 sessions I was pain free and could be more active. In hind sight I think I would have done better with a lot more treatments, but landed up coming back home to SA. But it was enough to get me going. I was basically pain free for 2 years until I became pregnant. I avoided severe exercises as I was too scared to test the boundaries, but I did garden and I dragged rocks around, which is actually a heavy workout. I would make sure I took Panado after my gardening session to ensure I didn't get too sore. You will do anything to avoid THAT pain again.

There were certain things I had to be very careful with. One of them is over-stretching. Another is rolling too long on a roller. I had to avoid doing any jumping activity as my calves would die the next day and frankly for the next week, so not worth it. I had to avoid sitting too long or standing too long or walking too far or exercising too long. Too much of anything really sucks. I can't walk too far or exert myself in any way, as you would for a competition. Such as swimming too fast or running, that is a guaranteed migraine. So I swim like an old lady and I walk like a duck and I ride around the block on my bike on a good day.

I have learnt what I like to do and how to do it within moderation. I have learnt what to do when I have the pain and who to go and see to help me get over the pain. I have learnt that the needles are king and the only thing that works for me. I have learnt that I love what I do and that I can get others to love the needles too.

Although the car accident was one of the worst experiences pain wise I have ever had, it was also one of the most important experiences I have had. If I had not had the car accident, I would not understand what my patients are going through. It is not in our head and we are not hypochondriacs. If we had no pain, we would not visit the doctors and keep going to different people in the hope someone will help us. Our headaches are real, the restless legs are real, and the aching and cramping are real. The fact that we can't sleep is real and makes us crankier. And when you feel as bad as you do, then yes, you would also feel depressed because everyone you go to does not understand what you are going through and all they want to do is put you on antidepressants, which frankly is not going to fix the problem. You feel misunderstood, confused and worst of all, the pain is still there and the handful of pain pills and other pills you are on, are not working.

So you sit stuck between a wall and a hard rock and cry some days, on the bad days, because, what am I going to do to get better and who is this person I have become?

But there is hope, because there are many Doctors and Physios out there who do know how you feel and do know what to do to help in getting you better, but you have to find them. I am currently learning a lot through the functional medicine group and the integrated health system. There are many medical people who are studying through them and they are helping chronic pain and chronic medical problems to return to normal. It is a really important movement that is taking place and I am pleased to say that I am part of this movement.

If I had not had this accident I would not have been taken along a path of self-discovery. This propportunity has made me interested in treating other patients who are also struggling with chronic pain and it has made me good at what I do. I have learnt many different techniques that I now use with my patients and there are some techniques I like way more than others and we will share these with you as we go along your journey of self-discovery and healing.

Chapter 3
Dry Needling, IMS and acupuncture

The dry needling was one of the first techniques that I really felt benefit with. I was introduced to this technique in my final year at university during one of our lectures. It intrigued me so that I attended my first course soon after. What I felt when those needles were placed in my body was amazing. This is how I explain it to my patients.

The needle works in three different ways. Firstly there is a foreign object being inserted into the body, which will create an activation of your immune system to heal the area, sending the soldiers to do their work. Inflammation will be created from the needle but this in itself is healing as there is an increase in blood flow and thus a removal of toxins. Secondly because the needle has two different metals on it, a silver part which is inserted into the body and a copper part which is wound around the silver part at the top (the handle) this will create a magnetic current.

I am sure many of you can remember standard 6 science, where you sent a current through a metal wire with copper wire bent around it. You then placed paper clips around this wire and sent a current through. It created a magnetic field which spun the paperclips all into the same direction. This is what happens in your body too. The blood is the current and the P factor which causes the Pain and the other chemicals that are heaped up and stuck in the muscle spasm and pain area are the paper clips, with the needle being the instigator of the magnetic current. When they are stuck into the body this magnetic current occurs and the stored chemical are removed from the area. As the needle is inserted one often gets a jump or twitch in the muscle. I often tell my patients that the muscle is jumping for joy. In science it is told that maximal contraction gives you maximal relaxation and this is the third phenomenon that has occurred.

The needles can have such a powerful effect that I have had patients enter my practice in a wheel chair because of pain and then walk out of there as if nothing was ever wrong with them. They all ask me if I have injected something into them, but it is just a needle with no fluid, hence why they call it dry needling. Wet needling is when you go to the doctor for an injection.

The needle itself is very thin. It has a sharp point like a pin would have, thus it does not cut the muscle when it enters like the injection needles do. It glides through the muscles. There are different length needles which enable us to reach the different depths of muscles. So in the thoracic area you would use a short needle to avoid complications such as pneumothorax. In the neck, depending on the thickness of the neck, one would use a slightly longer needle and in the buttock area where it is nicely padded, one would use an even longer needle. When inserting the needle you want to get all the way through the soft tissue until you hit bone again, so it is important to know what length to use as it can be dangerous if you do not know what you are doing or if you use the wrong length.

This technique is such a powerful technique that it can elicit an autonomic effect. One can experience the following effects and each patient is informed of these feelings before they are needled as well as after to remind them. Firstly, one will feel as if a train or bus has hit you for two days. You will have a feeling that you are bruised and have had a serious workout. Secondly, you can experience feelings of extreme happiness or sadness. You can become so tired that you may even fall asleep behind the wheel while driving. You can break out in an intense sweat or get goosing all over the body where the needles went in. You can cry for no reason when the needle is inserted as one stores emotions in the muscle spasms and when released so too will the emotion. I have often had patients who suddenly start to cry and when you ask if it is too painful, they say, they are feeling no pain, they don't know why they are crying. I have also had patients who suddenly start to shake. This is truly a wonderful reaction and I often tell my patients that we have just activated the parasympathetic mechanism of healing.

Then I tell them this story. When a buck is being chased by a lion, it runs and jumps for its life. If it does not get caught and the lion gives up, the buck will lie down on the grass have spasms/shaking throughout its body and when these spasms are finished, the buck will get up and carry on eating as if nothing has ever happened to it.

This happens to us too. When we have had a shock and the threat has passed we can start to shake. I experienced this after my dog bite injury. I had been walking my dog around the block with my son a few years ago. We were on our way home when a little sausage dog crawled out from under his fence and into the road to bark at my dog. It was standing there for a long time and I was watching a car coming along and I am convinced this person was texting on her phone. The car was so far away when this dog came into the road that I was sure she would see it. I was waving my arms and shouting at her and she just drove over the dog, both with the front and the back wheel. She pulled over to peer in her rear view mirror to see what had happened, while I ran to the dog. My son went hysterical and my dog was coming closer to see what was happening. I turned to tell my son to calm down as I was bending down towards the dog and at that moment the dog jumped up and locked its jaws onto my index finger. I got such a fright that I tried to shake the dog off and thus dislocated my finger which resulted in the dog releasing its hold. The finger was deformed and the blood was dripping off it.

The lady who had been watching all this pulled away and didn't even bother to help. I had the local community security car also watch everything that had happened and he at least offered some paper towel, but also left. I was mad that this lady who had created all this mess could just drive off like that. I know she knows that she was in the wrong. So I marched home with my dog and my son and went to the hospital with my mangled finger.

When I got to the hospital and was waiting for them to take me in, I experienced this shaking and knew exactly what it was. I had my shake and then when that was done I had a little personal chuckle. They needed to book me in for the night as they needed to set the joint and clean the wound as the dogs' teeth slid down the length of my finger muscle splitting it in half from the one little joint to the next. While I was lying in the hospital every nurse that came to evaluate me would ask what had happened. When I would say that a dog had bitten my finger, they would all ask if it was my dog that had bit my finger and I would reply "My Dog does not bite!" After about the third time I started to laugh about this as it reminded me of the Pink Panther:

The man was standing in the shop next to a dog and asked the Pink Panther "Does your dog bite?" To which the Pink Panther answered: "My dog does not bite." The man then bent down and the dog bit his hand, as he jumped back he said to the Pink Panther: "I thought you said your dog does not bite!" and the Pink Panther answered "That is not my dog!"

As for the dog, it had a broken leg which was also splinted and seems to me that the dog has recovered well. I am sure though that it also has stiffness of the joint just like I do.

I say to my patients that whatever the emotion or feeling that comes up, that it is quite possible that it can be from the needles and that they not worry, as it should pass by the next morning. Some symptoms though like shortness of breath should not be left as this is one of the signs of a pneumothorax. Blue lips, feeling anxious, struggling to breathe etc. Sometimes you will get a bruise from the needle and this will also pass.

When the needle is inserted into the body it will create a deep aching feeling. It really feels like you are exactly on the spot. It is actually more painful to massage the sore muscle than it is to stick a needle into it. Patients are usually sceptical when I say that until they have experienced the needle.

In our country we have many people who say it is against their religion to have the needles, which is why I want to explain the different between the dry needling and acupuncture. The technique has got nothing to do with religion. Dry needling is a westernized technique that was developed and there are books written on it to explain how it works and what it does scientifically. To break it down, we look for the tight bands that are found within the muscle, or we target known trigger points in specific areas for each muscle. The needle is then inserted in these bands or very specific trigger points which have been mapped out in these books. The needle needs to be put in exactly the right position to elicit the deep ache and feeling that the arm or leg is going to fall off from the ache. This then releases the muscle and you get instant increase in range of movement in the muscle which increases range of movement in the joint, decreases pain and improves strength.

I have had patients with frozen shoulders come for treatment and if it is caused by muscle spasm and the joint capsule is not tight, then the patient gets instant full use of the arm. Especially when the subscapularis muscle is released.

It is the most amazing technique to use and once you have experienced the benefits of it, then you will never use anything else. I have several patients who phone and say "You know how much I hate the needles, but I really think I need them." The good outweighs the bad tenfold.

Many physiotherapists dislike using the needles for several reasons; the main being that they are scared to cause more harm than good, a philosophy all good medical people adhere to. Others don't think that it is beneficial as it is too painful. Other still believe that there are other techniques that are better. In my opinion, there is nothing as powerful as needle therapy and I will always use it as the benefits I have experienced in my body indicate that for many it is the only appropriate technique.

When I went to the UK, they did not recognize my dry needling course and told me that I needed to do the acupuncture course if I wanted to use the needles on my patients. So I went and did the course. It is totally different to dry needling. The same needles are used, but they talk about meridians, Ying and yang (male and female) organs. Each meridian represents a different organ and runs along a specific path in the body. There are 10 meridians 5 male and 5 female. For instance the kidney meridian will start at the innersole of the foot and work its path upwards toward the inner knee and upwards further. This is one of the Ying meridians. They also look at your tongue and take your pulse and look in your eyes and make a decision as to which organ path is affected and stick needles in along the path.

The little weekend course I did was not complete enough for me to know everything about acupuncture, but what I have felt as I have experienced both techniques on my body, is that the acupuncture does not resolve the particular muscular problem as quickly as Dry needling does. I feel that both have merit and should have a positive effect as the needle will improve body function regardless of where it is inserted.

When I experience dry needling and the needle is inserted in the area that is causing the pain, the pain can go away instantly or take a day or two. If I have acupuncture and the needle is stuck in my legs or arms along a specific meridian for my buttock pain, then the legs and arms feel looser and the buttock stays the same. This empirical evidence indicates for me that Dry-needling is more potent to resolve the problem immediately. Perhaps the acupuncture is helping resolve the imbalance in the body and will take a lot longer to fix, but in this day and age, no one wants to wait that long to see results.

The third form of needling that I have experienced is IMS (intra-muscular stimulation). This technique is the best by far, but is the most painful. It requires some mental preparation before challenging oneself to IMS needling. I tell my patients that we are going to do extreme needling and as they are sport fanatics or have severe chronic pain and are desperate for improvement they will just have to endure the pain, as it is not for that long.

In this technique you needle the muscle on a stretch to get improved range, such as trying to do the split or need to get increased hamstring length to get a higher leg lift in sport. You also needle the whole body in a session. Each muscle gets many needles to release the entire muscle and the needles are pulled in and out to change the angle getting many muscle twitches. If you have a plunger then this is used.

The Physio needled every part of my body during my first IMS session in 45 minutes. After my session my entire body was stiff. I had to walk 20 minutes to the nearest train station and by the time I got to the station my legs and body had warmed up and the pain and stiffness was reduced. When I got home I took a warm bath and placed hot packs on my claves. The next day I felt so amazing it was unreal. I was loose for the first time in 10 years and felt I could do an aerobics session without a problem. The pliability of my skin on my arms had also changed so drastically that I kept touching my arms to feel the softness of the muscles and skin. It is truly the most amazing technique that I have had the privilege to experience and learn. It was also the technique that got me pain after only 6 sessions. I was pain free for two years as a result. The pain after my pregnancy has never been nearly as bad as the pain I experienced for 10 years and any recurrence of pain can be treated via needling.

Remember though, that if you are not responding to the needles, that you may have vitamin insufficiencies or other contributing factors and this will need to be resolved to improve your health. The needling releases the muscle, however if the pain is caused by a repetitive practice or the patient does not follow through with the required stretching and exercises the problem is likely to recur.

Chapter 4
Goal setting

Now you have read a part of my story and maybe you feel the same way I did; Confused, desperate, gatvol, irritated, tired, fat and frumpy and worst of all, still sore. So in this chapter I would like to get your brain to think about what it is you DO want, before I tell you how to get it.

I came across the following a few years ago and use it each year to determine what I would like to achieve and work on for the year. It's more than just a new year's resolution; it's a plan of action for the year. I now also use this with most of my patients as many of them have lost the fun in life and don't know what they want out of life, they are going through the motions of living and going to work and live with pain, misery and depression. This is a terrible position to be in but you can do something about it, because if your brain knows what you want out of life, then it goes out of its way to get it. If you just go through your daily actions without knowing what you want out of life, then you have to be happy with what life has dealt you.

I mention throughout the book all the things that have happened to me accidentally and as a result of decisions that I have made. By the end of 2014 I was feeling confused, lost and not enjoying life at all. Although I did my yearly goals I was not reaching them and this made me feel frustrated and irritated and I decided that I needed to take time out and really think about what was going on and why I was feeling like I did.

I spent 6 months with the guidance of an EFT (emotional freedom technique) practitioner working on different concepts and thinking about things. I took it a step further and added the goal setting chart to my preparation work for the weekly sessions, so that I knew what I wanted to tap about and this helped me to get clarity in my life and helped me move forward. I will explain in detail what EFT is in a later chapter, but when you are tapping on difficult situations or feelings, it is always better to do it with someone else as their insight can be very valuable, as they may see things totally differently to you as their experiences are different to yours. If you are seeing a Psychologist then use the EFT during your sessions to help move things faster.

Others are often gentler towards you than you are towards yourself. I often find that because I have experienced so many feelings of pain, frustration, irritation and depression, that when my patients tell me of a situation they have been through or going through I can empathize 100%. I know exactly how I felt and even if the situation is slightly different, because I have this plethora of feelings, I can imagine how I would feel if I was in their shoes. The little question one must also constantly ask, is WHY? If you just keep asking why, you come up finally with insight that is priceless and that is when the penny drops and you have your ah ha moment on why you do things a certain way or why you feel a certain way. This is the crux of the treatment. Once this happens, you heal and can move forward. The mind becomes crystal clear and you become motivated to do what you need to do to get better.

So with no further ado, let's delve into what you can do to change the way you think about life and to get your life back on track to not only have more fun, but to actually achieve things that you have always wanted to do.

How it works, is you take each area of the pie chart and allocate a number out of 10 indicating how happy you are with that specific area of your life. Zig Ziglar refers to it slightly differently and calls it your life wheel.

Thus 0 is dreadful and 10 is great.

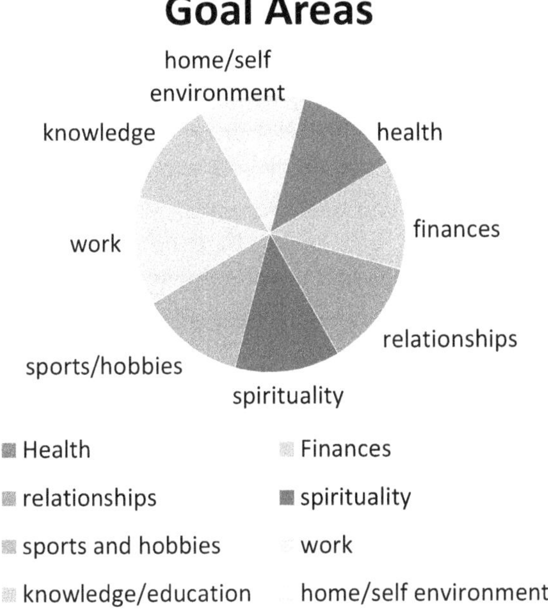

Now you write down everything you would like to achieve in each of the areas, in detail. See below for examples. Always try to write in the positive and not use negative terminology, as your brain tends to get stuck on the negative.

1: Health:

What I have discovered about the health section, is that if your health is compromised, then you will find it hard to do any of the other areas as you cannot concentrate or exercise or work hard or think outside the box if you are not feeling well. So please make sure that this section is considered the most important area if you are sick, and that you focus on this area and perhaps one other when you start working towards your goals.

Out of the 6 fundamental factors, which we cover in another chapter, your thoughts need to be positive to be able to achieve anything that you write down in the goal area, however the diet is the most important aspect that can change the way you look, feel and think. It can reverse illness and get your DNA to reboot and function properly. Thus do not take this area lightly and if you do not know what to do to get what you want, make sure you get yourself a coach to help you move forward.

So my goals that I wrote down in my health section are just an idea as to what you can work towards. Please add other goals if you have others.

a: I would like to weight 52Kg
b: I would like to have enough energy to walk/swim/Cycle as a form of exercise
c: I would like to feel refreshed daily, by having a great nights' sleep every night
d: I want to have clear energized skin with even colour tones of brightness. (instead of writing "no dark circles under my eyes")
e: I would like to have a flat stomach
f: I would like to have supple muscles and soft pliable skin and muscles (instead of no pain and no headaches)
i: I want to feel like I am having fun all the time and to enjoy doing the things I take part in.

2: Finances:

Now I am not a financial advisor, but I did this exercise and I can tell you it has made the worlds difference in my life.

In 2015 I changed my bank but could only move my cheque account and credit card account over and had to leave the house bond and money market at the other bank. I only lasted 6 months at the new bank before I had to return to the original bank, because electronic banking is not seamless. Each month my debit orders would go off and because I did not know how much money was going off at the beginning of each month, I wouldn't have enough money in the account and would land up going into the red. As it takes 4 days for your money to clear when transferring from the one bank to the other, my debit orders would then be rejected and additional bank fees incurred. I have never felt so stressed out. I never had the problem when all my accounts were at the same bank, as I would transfer from the money market directly and immediately over to the cheque account as soon as I saw the funds were running low. The new bank never sent me credit card statements, so I never knew when or what was due and the interest accumulated and my stress accumulated and in the end I told the bank to cancel my accounts as it took them the entire 6 months to resolve the issue and then wanted to know why I was leaving.

I felt overwhelmed with the stress of not knowing how much money I needed to have in my bank account at the beginning of each month to ensure all the debit orders that went off where covered. I decided that I was spending too much money and that I needed to see where I could cut back on the spending and go through the debit orders to see if I could cancel or change some.

So I firstly closed my account and got all my eggs back into one bank. Then I sat down and went through all the debit orders that went off and wrote them all down and added them all up, so that I knew exactly how much money went off each month and I could be prepared well in advance for the debit orders to go off. This was amazing, as I started seeing that there were debit orders that were too expensive and others that were pointless. I then went through each one and stopped them or reduced them and I was so much more in control of my finances and it made me feel as though my year's goal was beginning to take shape. I think this is vital to do regularly as you are constantly signing more debit orders that creep the expenses up even though it is only R100 here and R75 there. It all adds up at the end of the month.

I sat and calculated how much money I needed to earn a month and worked it back to how many patients I needed to see per day/week. This helped me relax in the quiet weeks as long as I was on target for the month. I could work out what I would like to earn, save and spend each month knowing that I could achieve it.

I now keep track of my expenses and debit orders on a spread sheet that I go through monthly and add all the figures in. By the time the end of the tax year arrives, I am ready to meet with the accountant as everything has been kept up to date and all I need to wait for are the certificates from the companies. It is very useful to be organized like this.

a: I would like to earn R......./month
b: I would like to have low expenses not more than R.....
c: I would like to save Rx each month/by the end of the year. You can tie this in to tax the free savings or your retirement investments
d: I would like to find an alternative income outside of my work
e: I would like to find a financial advisor who will be able to help me set up a good retirement and get my money to make more money.

3: Relationships:

There are many books out there that can help you in this area. Some of my favourites are *"Personality plus" by Florence Littauer,* this book talks about the different personalities and what their likes and dislikes are. If you know what type of person your spouse is then it is easier to deal with them. This book explains the Choleric/melancholy/Sanguine/Phlegmatic personalities that I touched on in the first chapter. There is a questionnaire that you complete and this tells you your personality type. It points out your weaknesses and your strengths and helps you understand your colleagues you may be having trouble with, or why you are struggling with your family members. Once you know how to spot a personality, you will be able to identify which personality your friends, family etc. are and this could be quite fun to do.

The other book that helped a lot was *"The 5 love languages" by Gary Chapman*; here he speaks about how different people feel loved and validated. At the beginning of each relationship you tend to do all the different love languages as you want to impress the other person, but after a while you no longer do this as you just tend to do the ones that you like. The five love languages are gifts, quality time, positive affirmations, deeds done and touch. So if you are a gift person, you will often give gifts to your spouse. If they are not a gift person, then the gifts won't really make them feel loved. If you are a touch person, you will always give hugs or touch people on their shoulders or arms as a means of endearment. If you are not getting your quota of hugs in then you feel unloved. The books talks about an empty love tank. This empty love tank results in you finding this love in other places. This is why it is so important to make sure you know what your spouses' love language is, so that the family is always happy and kept close.

When the love tank is empty you may hear them complain that you do not keep the house clean or that you don't spend enough time with them or that you are never available, or you don't give enough hugs or you are always complaining about the things they are doing. The thing that they are usually complaining about is usually their love language that has not been fulfilled, so they don't feel that you love them and their love tank is empty.

This is easy enough to resolve. By doing the test at the back of the "*The 5 love languages*" book you can find out which love language each person in the house is and even your friends, and then you can make a point of speaking their love language and before you know it, you and they will be feeling far more validated and loved and you will feel good and they will feel good and things will be easier in the house. It is said when you feel loved, you will be able to concentrate better and perform better.

I have this patient who has global pains and some of the problems she experiences are that her hips are too painful for her to sit on the floor and enjoy a meal in a specific restaurant. She also has swelling of her fingers and is unable to wear her wedding ring. So when I suggested that she set herself goals and make sure that her husband is included in celebrating them when she achieves them, she sat down with him, explained what she wanted to achieve and the two of them came up with the following ideas.

When she is able to sit cross legged on the floor for a period of time, they will go out and celebrate at the restaurant where they have to sit on the floor. When her fingers are not swollen and she is able to get her wedding ring on, then they will go out for a romantic meal and ceremoniously put her ring back on. These little mile stones are important to celebrate and they create peace and a sense of love and achievement.

Each person is different and there is no wrong way to reward yourself. I like to buy myself gifts when I reach certain milestones or achieve goals. So when my menstrual cycle returned back to normal, (who thought you would be excited about menstruating) I went and bought myself a beautiful rose quartz pendant and matching ring. When I had harvested my eggs and my friend was pregnant with triplets I purchased an amazing oil painting that I sit for hours admiring. When she lost them I bought both of us a moonstone pendant surrounded by an angel, a rose and a butterfly symbolizing the positions the babies were in the womb. Although this was not a goal achieved, it was to remember them by and it has become one of my favourite pieces to wear. It is now symbolic of what I have been through physically and emotionally and becomes a symbol of determination.

When I got my first pay check ever, I went out and bought myself a pearl ring with a diamond set over the top, a stunning piece. This was a fond memory and I felt very grown up. Every time I wear these items, it takes me back to that memory and it is good to remember. I am stopping and smelling the roses.

My son knows me so well. He always asks me what he can get for my birthday, either jewellery or clothes that he can buy with my money (he is only 9 now), because if he goes to the only shop he can get to, tuck shop, then he can only get me a chocolate or snack which is the only thing he can afford and he knows I prefer the jewellery. In children all the love languages are relatively even as we get older we have one or two that become more dominant.

If you are not a reader or do not like to listen to CD books, then it could be valuable to attend a relationship seminar. I took my husband to one called Imago therapy. The interesting concept that they used was to ensure that you listen to your spouse. So you are asked to tell a story about how you feel and they must repeat back exactly what you said. Often they change the words, changing the entire meaning of the sentence you said. You are then requested to stop them and tell them that that is not what you said. You repeat the sentence and they must again repeat what you said until they have the exact same meaning you told them in the first place. This gives such clarity and there can be no misunderstanding.

I have used this technique with my patients when they tell me their story. At the end I say, "what I hear is that ……… and this is how you feel……..'' if I have not got it right, they add to the sentence or retell the story until I understand where they are coming from, so that I can help them get better. I also point out all the areas they are complaining of again. This gives us both an idea of what is going on, as I can explain why they are like they are and what we are going to do together to improve the situation. I have wonderful compliance.

No one is taught how to keep a relationship going, you follow from example. You will tend to do what your parents did and if you didn't have very good role models, then it makes it rather difficult to have a good relationship. There are so many tools available to you today that it is possible to find another role model or different viewpoints to the one you were brought up with. You get counsellors, Google, books, friends who have great relationships and so the list goes on. The books I mentioned have been pivotal in my relationships and that many patients have found them very useful in theirs.

So what would you like?

a: I would like to keep a close understanding relationship with my son
b:I would like to keep a close understanding relationship with my partner.
c: I would like to have a few close friends that I can do fun things with.
d: I would like to do fun things at least once a month with my family (weekend away, medieval fayre, nice dinner out, movies, go for a bike ride etc.)

4: Spirituality

In this section, I don't necessarily mean going to church. I have found that if you spend quiet time being grateful for what you have and think about what you would like out of life and go through the goal wheel we are discussing in this chapter you will achieve amazing results.

When I was in the UK I would spend 10min each morning planning my day down to the hour. I would see a patient every 30min in the UK and a new patient would take an hour, now I see my patients one per hour because of the nature of their problems. I would spend 2 min every morning at 10am just sitting and becoming quiet and each night as I was falling asleep I would run through everything that I was grateful for. It was actually so amazing how things would fall into place and happen with no effort at all.

I remember I was organizing a course and I needed to have 12 people on the course to be able to afford the lecturer. It was 2 weeks before the course and I was still 5 people short. I really didn't want to cancel the course as it was something that I really wanted to do. So I spent the morning running through my day in my head and asking that 3 people must call to book onto the course. As the day progressed, it was not even lunch time yet, when 3 people called almost straight after each other and booked to come on the course. I was overjoyed as there were only 2 still needed. That night I went through what I was grateful for. The next morning I did the same and said that I wanted to have another 2 people call to book on the course and believe it or not, two people called that day again before lunch time and the course was a huge success. Again that night I went through everything that I was grateful for.

It did not stop there. I remember getting on the bus to go home and the rain bucketing down. I had no umbrella and was not in the mood to walk home in the rain. So as I was driving along I thought that it would really be nice if the rain would stop long enough for me to just walk home. Like magic as I got off the bus, the rain stopped and as I walked in the front door it started again, my foot even got wet the timing was so perfect.

We underestimate the power of gratitude and the power of prayer and becoming quiet. You need to have a balance between work, play and rest. Prayer and quiet falls in the rest aspect and without balance in your life you do not have things handed to you on a golden platter.

When I started learning how to become quiet and meditate/clear my mind, it was very difficult and I felt guilty for sitting around doing nothing, I also got very bored. My aunt used to come and visit every Saturday at my folks home and spend the night. One Saturday we decided that we would begin to meditate. I have a few relaxing CDs and guided meditation CDs and each Saturday we would put a CD on. 5 Minutes into the CD I had had enough and was fidgeting as I was uncomfortable, but I sat still as my aunt was deep in meditation. Even the cat liked it and would run into the room when we were getting ready and he would sit there the entire time. I thought it was rather strange, but my aunt told me that the cat was intuitive and knew exactly what we were doing.

It took me a year before I could drift away into quietness and sit for the entire CD only waking when I heard the CD spin to a stop. I think my aunt had been doing this for years as she explained to me several times how it worked and what to do. I was blessed to have her help me through the process. I gained so much insight and felt rejuvenated and many things happened positively. Some people feel uncomfortable with the word meditation. Then think of it as prayer or relaxation. But it has been shown to improve your parasympathetic response in your body which is the healing response. Your sympathetic nervous system is the flight fight response and we are all over-active in this area with all the stress we experience and the long working hours we are determined to do. It is actually very important do be able to activate your parasympathetic response and this is one of the ways you can do this.

There are different ways to activate it, you can do deep breathing. You can go for a massage. You can do Chi Gung or Tai chi, you can sit outside in your garden and take in the beauty with no talking. You can go for a quiet walk in nature. You can do Yoga. The important thing is to become quiet and think about nothing, or to only take in what is beautiful around you. I like to sit at my fish pond and watch them swim. You go into a trance staring at them swimming around. If my son is there, who has the inability to be quiet; I tell him that it is quiet time and get about 5 minutes of silence out of him. This will improve as the time goes by and he learns how to sit quietly like I had to with my aunt.

When you improve your quiet time and find that balance of rest hard, work hard, play hard, you will create infinite possibilities of positive things happening in your life.

This is very important to be able to do this aspect of the wheel, so what would you like to be able to do?
a: I would like to meditate once a week for 1 hour
b: I would like to plan my day with a prayer and 10min quiet time
c: I would like to feel more in tune with my life and things around me.
d: I would like to remember to be grateful every night when I go to bed
e: I want life to feel easy and things to come easily to me
f: I want to teach my son to find balance

5: Sport and hobbies

Many of the patients whom I have been treating have found that they have not been able to do any form of sport of hobbies, either because they have too much pain and thus flare up the pain by doing exercises, or they do not have the energy to the do the hobby or sport because they have adrenal fatigue. During my time of goal setting and soul searching, I was thinking about the fact that life was not a great deal of fun at that moment in time. I was at a loss as to what was fun. I was setting up goals and going through the motion of what I wanted out of life, but thinking that I did not know what I actually wanted to do. I didn't have energy to do anything and thus didn't want to do anything. I felt irritated with myself because I usually get so much done and achieve even more than normal, but over the past few years it felt like I was not doing anything that was fun. I was not even achieving anything.

So I sat down and thought for a good number of days: "When was the last time that I can remember having fun?" I came to the conclusion that it was at school. I then thought: "What was I doing that was fun?" I came to the conclusion that I enjoyed doing sport and music and singing and being creative. I then asked: "Why was it fun?" and "what about that activity makes it fun?" I came to the conclusion that being active with people is fun. If I break down the activity, I found that I like to be doing things, I like to be active and I like it when I am good at doing it and people notice and compliment me on the thing I was doing. My love tank is being filled.

My next question was: "What am I doing now that would fall in the category of having fun?" I came to the conclusion that my belly dancing was "Fun" and my treatments were Fun and my gardening was fun. So my next question I asked was: "If these are supposed to be fun, then why am I not having fun and it feels like it is a chore to do the fun things?" and my conclusion to this was: "Because I have adrenal fatigue I am not having fun, because I get too tired." So I then turned it around and said: "If I continue with these activities that are supposed to be fun, I will know that I am better when I actually enjoy going to class or enjoy doing the activity." This really made me feel much better and when I did feel that the class was fun I then made a point of making some pretty Belly outfits to celebrate the fact that I had achieved a goal.

With chronic pain one really does struggle to do any form of exercise, but you can really break it down to manageable levels, by focusing on a stretching program and walking, aiming to get your steps up to 10 000 per day. If you are unable to do 10 000 steps because of pain/fatigue or anything else, start with 2000 steps and each week or so increase the amount of steps taken. Also make sure you are attending your treatment to help you get looser and less painful so you can progress your exercises. There are also some basic exercises that you can do which take a few minutes, but strengthen your back, stomach, legs and arms. These I often recommend to my patients.

They are wall push-ups, Pilates sit-ups, Bridging and squats. 10 of each and as you are able to do them easier, increase the repetitions and voila you will see changes. One of my patients' whom I have given these exercises to, has been doing them for several months now and he informed me that he has started to get definition in his legs. Furthermore, he no longer has back or neck pain and is able to continue with his program on his own with a check-up from time to time. This is a man who had permanent severely debilitating headaches and back pain for 30 years of his life and within 10 months he is pain free from focusing on these simple goals. He has also been able to increase his steps from barely making 2000 to 6000 and he has progressed his exercises from 10 to 20 repetitions. He eats well and sleeps well and has goals set up for the year, so has purpose in his life. He is ecstatic and so am I.

So what do you want?
a: I would like to cycle 10km with ease
b: I would like to be more flexible and better with my dancing
c: I would like to sing and play the piano again
d: I would like to improve my sight reading for the piano
e: I would like to enjoy my gardening regularly and help others to have a beautiful garden.

6: Knowledge and education

When I was at university I read a book by Robert Kiyosaki. He has written so many, but think it may have been "*Rich dad poor dad*." In this book he said that at the end of each month, you must take your salary and pay 10% to further your education in a field outside your field of work. Then you must take 10% and put it away for pension and then you must take 10% and give it away to charity. After reading this book I made a point of each year or so picking something different to do.

The first 2 years I did singing in the form of light opera, then I did a year of art, how to draw with pencil and shadowing. I then did a year on modelling and how to walk the cat ramp. Then I did photography, a garden design course and spent the next few years getting my garden to look fantastic. I lectured in my physio field to qualified physiotherapist and assisted on another physio course for about 2 years. I did dog school for 3 years and now have an amazing dog. I started doing belly dancing as a form of recreation and I like it so much I have continued with it. I am interested in going back to singing and back to playing the piano and learn how to sight read music. Shocking as I already have my Grade 7 piano.

I am interested in doing a birding course to identify birds and I am interested in learning more in my field of healing and am writing this book as I feel I need to share my knowledge. I have done a course on stock trading and did a year stock trading with a mentor. I have done a course on the EFT (emotional freedom technique) and found it so useful I did all the other courses and the matrix re-imprinting and now use it in my work. I have done a nutritional course through Paul Check and the Check Institute and his information is also so valuable I use it in my daily practice. I am now doing a course on functional medicine to better my knowledge. I have joined a continued education program where I get a book each month on self-development in a range of different areas that I would not have chosen for myself. A lot of information that I share with my patients comes from these books, which then become a part of who you are. These books also gave me the belief that I could also write a book.

So each year I do something and if I like it I continue and when I get tired of it or the course is finished or the goal has been achieved, then I move on to the next challenge. By doing this you achieve many things and have a large background of information to talk from. Thus when you are in a social environment, you are able to talk about many different things and surely come up with something that is common in the person whom you are talking to. This makes for very interesting conversations, it also makes you far more positive and entertaining. I enjoy conversation and learning about others and their interests. The information also gives you wisdom to draw from and it has helped many people get insight into problems they are experiencing and are then able to overcome.

I was really impressed to hear how this has rubbed off on a number of people whom I have mentioned it to. One of the ladies at Belly dance was telling me how this has inspired her to go do a singing course and her daughter is going with. She said it helped her make a decision to leave her current work and to start her own company which she had wanted to do for a long time.

If you think about it, your entire school career was set up to teach you specific knowledge. When you went to university you were taught more in a specific area. But when you qualify or finish school, what do you do to improve yourself? In the medical field and some other fields, it has become law for us to continue our education in our field; otherwise we lose our license to treat. However there are many people out there that do nothing to further their knowledge, which means you stagnate where you are.

As Jim Dornan says, leaders are readers.

He also says, what gets measured gets improved. I have not had the privilege to meet Jim, and unfortunately he has passed away, but I have listened to many of his talks on CD and love his way of explaining and wisdom he brings through.

None of the knowledge you gain is wasted. I go through the goal setting list with my patients, then in the last section where you do garden and home environment, I offer to design their garden for them, to create a haven for them to go home to. This has been a new challenge for me and is bringing such fun to my life. I then take many pictures of my garden and the new gardens, using my photographing skills. My dog is so well trained that the patients love him and he has become part of my treatment room and gives them well needed love but will also go lie down when told to do so. Dogs have been used to smell cancers and there are studies that show they improve general well-being and they are a great stress reliever.

Each book I have read has added to my self-growth and it has been an amazing journey. As mentioned in many sections, there is always a book that has inspired me to think outside the box and to understand a difficult situation and make it into a propportunity. What do I mean by a propportunity, the book I read *"Living your life through pathological positivity."* the author Paul H Jenkins, writes about how we must try and see each problem in its most positive light and how you can change this problem into an opportunity, thus creating a new word, called a propportunity. I absolutely love this word. I use it often with my patients' as the pain they are experiencing is not a bad thing, as this journey of pain is teaching a bucket load of things, from patience on how to handle pain, to what kind of pain it is and so the list goes on, what is your pain telling you and what did you learn out of the situation. My pain led me down the path to become a physiotherapist who specializes in chronic pain and I am able to help a lot of people who previously had no hope and had been living with pain for many, many years. So what is your propportunity teaching you?

The other thing I have learnt from reading and listening to books is that you will be the same person in the next 5 years than you are today, except for the people you hang around with or meet, the books you read and the things you listen to. What does this mean? If you read books on a specific topic, let's take the self-improvement books we have been talking about, after 2 years of reading 20 min per day, you will gain insight from different perspectives that are not purely your own. Your tolerance of others foibles and habits will increase and you will become a kinder more interesting person. Unfortunately to become an expert requires 10 000 hours of exposure, training and application.

If you read a book on garden designing and plants, and you apply this knowledge to a garden where you can experience the results of a well-designed plan you will know more than most of your neighbours. What would you like to know more of and become good at? What knowledge do you want to gain or what in your life do you want to improve? We often ask many people questions on what we should be doing when we are experiencing problems, but are the people we are asking actually experts in the field and do they have your best interest at heart? You should be asking the experts and if you do not know any experts then go and find experts in books or CDs that you can buy at a reasonable price and start teaching yourself.

What I have found to be very useful is getting audio books. These books are easy to listen to while you are driving, and they are easy for your kids to listen to. They get exposed to good books and good advice and they may even become better rounded people. My son age 9 loves listening to the Emotional IQ audio book I got him and has listened to it several times already. How many children of that age have read that book? If I notice he is struggling with certain issues at school or elsewhere, then I track down the audio book I think may help him and give it to him as a surprise present. Firstly he loves getting presents and secondly considering he loves listening to stories when he goes to bed, he is quite happy to pop the book in and listen to what it has to say. Some of the stories enthral him so, that he is most willing to listen to it a number of times. I may have said exactly the same things, but it becomes part of you when you hear it from someone else or read it for yourself. It's almost as if you have been talking to yourself and agreeing with what you have to say.

So when we talk about where you are with your knowledge and education, one must think of what you would like to improve in yourself and perhaps what you would like to learn outside of your field of expertise and then what you need to learn in your field of expertise to improve the service you offer. With Google at the tips of your fingers, it makes it a lot easier to find the education you need or the experts that can guide you in getting the right books you need to read.

So jot down a few things you would like to try out and learn more about, both in your field of work as well as out.

a: I would like to attend a birding course on how to identify birds
b: I would like to know more in the medical field in functional medicine
c: I would like to go through the health DVDs I already have
d: I would like to teach myself to sight read music.

7: Work

Many of my patients who come see me suffer from working too hard and too many hours, feeling the stress of deadlines and feeling obliged to work all hours of the day and night just to get the work done. This is not right as it causes severe problems both with health and relationships. There needs to be a balance of working hard, playing hard, rest hard and you cannot get the balance if you are working all hours of the day and night.

You need to put your foot down and only work the hours you are being paid for. Yes on occasion you may need to work a few hours extra, but this should not be the norm.

When I was newly qualified I worked in a physio practice seeing 35 patients per day at 4 different places. When I signed up for the job, my working hours were 8-5 with an hour lunch. When I got there on the first day I had a new patient at 8 am for a neck treatment and at 8h15 I had a second new patient also for a neck treatment. It is not possible to treat a patient in 15 minutes as there is way too much to do with them and the evaluation takes 20 min if you do a proper evaluation on a simple patient. It can take up to an hour to evaluate a difficult patient. So needless to say I could not go against my conscience and only treat them for such a short period of time.

Luckily I had 6 cubicles to myself and could spread the patients and spend 10min with each person while the others had either needles in or electronic equipment working on them, but I felt stressed, and got 2 hours behind with my treatments and the people would complain about the fact that they would have to sit and wait for me to get to them. It got so bad that I would work through my lunch hour just to catch up and landed up working till 7 pm every night just to finish the patients who had been booked. So this resulted in the secretary booking patients for me during my lunch hour as well as after 5 pm. When I approached my boss, requesting that she pay me after hour rates as I was working more than my standard hours required, she turned around and told me that she didn't have money to do that as she was still paying off the machines she had bought.

I felt offended and only lasted 4 months there. I also discovered that she was spending money on importing Persian cats from America. She was paying me a very small salary and when I work out conservatively what I brought into the practice, my salary was only a few days' worth of work, far from the typical norm of 40-50% of what a physio writes. Mind you this was the longest anyone had lasted there. Some people left after the first day there.

When I told her that I was unable to stay after 5 pm the one day, because I had to fetch a friend from work as their car was broken, she was furious. She told me that she was not going to stay as she was not able to leave her kids standing on the side of the road at school waiting for her and because I had no life and I was not married and didn't have children, I must work. Well I didn't stay after 5pm and it was her problem, as I had told the secretary at the beginning of the day that I was not able to stay late. I also had to work every second weekend and when I did work the weekends, I would start at 6am and only finish at 6pm. I was knackered and didn't have time to go to the toilet, so I landed up with constipation and severe abdominal pains. Also I got a sinus infection that lasted for more than two weeks and I have suffered from sinus problems since then.

She used to tell me if I had already treated the patient 20 sessions with no results to just ask the Dr for another referral to get another 20 treatments. She made me store the needles in an envelope for each patient and have to re-use them. The problem I had with this was that I couldn't remember who the patients were, because I was seeing so many I could not keep track. At the end of the day I had to get the secretary to jog my memory as to which patient it was and she would have to describe the patient until I could remember who it was and what I did with them, so that I could write what I had done with them. So I felt super stressed and my body was sore and tired. My weekends off I spent all Saturday sleeping and walked around moping on Sunday.

I hated working there and started to hate being a physio, because I was earning so little and working so hard it was ridiculous. To make matters worse, I had a second job from 7h30 at night to 10pm treating boarding school boys, just to earn more money. I did get something good out of this though. I learnt how I didn't want to work and how I didn't want to be treated or treat patients. I had so many patients who often had the same problems meaning I could try a range of different techniques out and see which one worked the best and the fastest. This meant I would then use the best technique from the word go and get great results much faster. The Dry needling was one of them.

So now I treat my patients one per hour and take my lunch. I work to the time and try never to be late, because I know how much I hate to wait for an appointment, so try to never keep my patients waiting. I love what I do, and have time to fetch the kids in the afternoon and do homework with them (he does homework and I cook). Now that my energy is back I can walk around the block and do my sport (belly dancing) which is part of getting my balance in my life. I never want to go back to working all day and hating what I do, because my patients would feel the difference and that is not what I want to offer. I want to walk the talk. I can't expect you to do all these things if I am not doing them too.

So what are you doing that is compromising your health. What can you do to resolve this situation?

I had a patient who became very ill and for 3 years I kept telling her that she needed to change her job as it was making her very sick. She is a programmer who works to deadlines, but the work made the deadlines literally impossible to reach in normal working hours, so they would be forced to work till 1am or 2am each morning, go home to wake again at 6 am to be back at work at 8am and work till the next morning. The work refused to pay them over time, stating that they would be able to put their over-time hours in when the project was finished and then get time off. However, when the project was finished the company would quickly close the account and tell them that it was too late to put in the over-time and that they couldn't take time off because the next project was beginning the next day.

She worked like this for many years. She got severe adrenal fatigue that she is still struggling to recover from 2 years down the line, after resigning from the work. No other company wants to hire her because of the adrenal fatigue and worrying that it will be a liability for them and that she will take too many days off sick leave. She gained a lot of weight, became depressed, couldn't stay awake at work and had pain everywhere. But no one at work cares and now that she is sick no one wants to hire her. She has been unable to get work now for about a year and has had the time to heal her body. Recently she was accepted in a new position and hopefully this time round she will know better.

I get furious when I hear about things like this, and say to my young patients who are still eager to start working: "Start how you mean to end!'" if you want to be a workaholic then fine, but don't cry when the wheels fall off the bus. If you tell your boss that you are only available till 5pm or 4pm when you are supposed to finish work anyway, they will never ask you to work extra, because you told them in the beginning you can't. You should also not feel guilty about saying no.

When I started working from home, because I had a little baby and working at the hospital was not working out for me, I thought it was great and would book patients any time they wanted to come. The problem with that was that no one wanted to come in the middle of the day when it was easy and convenient to see them. They all wanted to come at the end of the day when it was bathing time and feeding time for my baby. I would have to bath him in 1 min flat while the patients were driving in to park and walking up the pathway. He would have to feed himself and put himself to bed. I would get the patients to read bedtime stories to him, and I felt terrible doing it. As he got older he would start to cry and ask me when I was going to spend time with him.

It became difficult to treat patients because I would have a crying baby wanting my attention and me feeling frustrated and irritated with the whole situation. So I stopped and decided to change the whole situation. I told my patients that I was no longer available in the afternoons and would start at 7am to compensate for those who had to go to work far and be there early. To my surprise everyone was happy to compromise and come at the allotted time slots and I had more time to spend with Vincent and read to him and put him in bed and sit with him while he ate. He was happy, I was happy and my patients got the benefit of having a calm physio and a calm baby, a win for everyone.

What do you want from work?

a: Work my working hours and no over-time
b: Work close to home or from home
c: Have a kind boss who is flexible when I need to meet Dr appointments or take care of my family
d: Work flexible hours
e: Get noticed for what I do and praised for doing good work
f: get paid well for what I do and get promoted easily

8: Home and self-environment

This is something I added after a while of doing the goal wheel. This is a different one, but as I notice that very few people actually have nice gardens or dress well, I feel it is something one needs to do.

Because I have done a gardening course I offer my patients an extra service of designing their garden for them. My garden is exquisite. I say this every day as I leave to fetch my son or come home and drive into the driveway. My patients when they arrive take their time coming up the path as they stop to enjoy the view. If I treat them on their side they spend their time looking out the window admiring the dragon flies and butterflies and birds and the fabulous garden. Best of all, everyone comments on how nice the garden looks and how they would love to have one too. This is why I offer the garden design to them.

This all came about when Vincent asked if he could earn extra money. He asked if he could treat my patients instead of me and then he could get paid for the work and not me. I told him that this was not possible as he has not studied physio and that he would not know what to do. To which he informed me that he watches what I do and that it does not look too hard and that he is sure he could do it just as well as I do. I had a chuckle and everyone else too and we scratched our head as to what he could do instead.

We came up with an idea to sell the fly catcher plants that had multiplied, which made him very happy, and within a short period of time he had sold all the plants and wanted to know what next. So we walked through the garden for inspiration and he started looking at it with new eyes and asked me if we could make babies from the plants in the garden like we did the fly catchers. This is how his nursery started. Then to help him sell his plants, I offered to design the gardens for my patients and then provide them with the plants from Vincent's nursery at a really good price. This means everybody wins. Vincent makes a profit, the patients get a stunning garden that they actually plant themselves using their own gardener. This means that they spend a lot less than if they got a landscaper in to design their garden and they have the pleasure of accomplishing it themselves over time.

I did this for a few of my patients already and the comments are all the same. They love their garden and many people ask them who helped them with the garden. When the people are told they did it by themselves, I am sure they feel boosted by the wonderful compliments as I do. One of my ladies said that she spends less money each month because she only needs one gardener instead of two. She had two gardeners full time because she wanted them to make it look nice, but all they did was cut the grass and weed but did not do anything else. So it never looked different from before. We went with a plan and hired a skip to get rid of the rubbish and started working with a plan. The garden transformed under her watchful eye to her amazement. We made paths throughout her garden, so she could walk through it and admire it. She has used this to her advantage by walking through her garden every evening until she has finished walking her 10 000 steps. She feels empowered and loves what she sees and best of all, because she wanted her garden to be an edible garden, she is picking apples and lemons and pears and berries and loving every minute of it: Food for the soul.

When you have a pretty home and garden, you want to be home. Your animals want to be home. My cats do not leave my garden. There are too many bushes and birds and things to entertain them. When I work with my patients I watch my cats walk up and down my paths and go and lie under the different bushes. Each cat has his favourite bush and when I walk my patients out I point out my cats to them enjoying the sun.

This is what I mean by home environment. This includes your house itself. Is it sunny and welcoming, or is it cluttered with rubbish. De-clutter, open it up and clean it out, if you do not know how, find someone who does or likes to do it. You may even have a family member that can come and help you. Clean your home every year. Go through the cupboards and get rid of all the old broken things or things you no longer wear and fix what you want to keep.

Over the holidays I went through my garden and fixed all the cracked and broken statues and then I repainted them all, so that they stand out in the garden again and look like new. I went through my cupboards and repacked them and threw away anything that was broken, or fixed it. I am now on the mission to help my cats feel happier, as a new kitten arrived in December which has caused my cats to start marking their territory all over the house. So now we incorporate play therapy and ensure they have many high places in the house to escape to and feel safe. Everyone in the house must feel that the home is homely. You must want to go home, not avoid going home.

When I talk about self-environment I mean how you dress and wear your hair and do your makeup. It has been said that it takes 30seconds to make a first impression. This is before you have even opened your mouth and greeted the person. So what kind of an impression do you want to leave?

As a physio we mostly work in T-shirt and shorts with takkies, or a uniform, which are mostly long pants with a golf shirt or shorts with a golf shirt. I used to work in T-shirt and shorts with takkies. I never really thought about my appearance until I went to a business seminar. Here I was very much aware of how well the people dressed and how good they looked. All the previous courses I had attended were with other physios who dressed the same, so it had never crossed my mind to dress differently.

After this seminar I decided that I needed to get some pretty business dresses. So I went to a boutique and asked the lady to help me find a business dress that would make me look as pretty as the image of mini mouse. She took two dresses off the rack and I looked at them with trepidation. But when I put them on, it was exactly what I had in mind and I bought them immediately. It was some time later when my sister in law mentioned that she was studying fashion design and colour and style analysis and asked if she could use me as a model that my eyes started to open to what she was talking about. She went through my cupboard and threw away half my clothes because they were the wrong colour for me. I had pretty much got my style right but because I was getting the style in the wrong colour, people would ask me if I was tired or sick. Some people are not able to wear black or lime green or orange and so the list goes on.

Yes I was tired and sick, but I didn't want to look tired and sick. So I followed her advice and added a few pretty belts under the chest and when I went to the shops to buy clothes I would stick to the colour swatch I carry in my bag. The very next day when I went to the hospital, the nursing staff stopped me and asked me to come show them what I had on. They then asked me to turn around slowly so they could admire the new look. The one nurse asked me: "What have you done differently, you still dress smart, but now you look really nice," to which I told them the whole story.

It is really amazing what you can do with a simple dress, by just adding a belt or pretty little shoes, that are still comfortable and the right accessories or my pretty pink necklace and other gems I have collected over the years. You always look nice and everyone wants to know where I am going. My answer to that is I am going to work and must always look good, because your first impression counts and I am a professional business woman and not a slob.

So I say to my patients that when they have reached certain goals that they should put this on the list of rewards. This has been one of the things I have done that has impacted me the most. I get many compliments on a daily basis just on what I am wearing, this alone make you feel on top of the world as it is nice to be complimented.

What do you need to change in your home?

a: change cat scratching posts to hold more cats and be higher
b: Play with cats to stop them spraying in the house
c: Finish the swimming pool in the back garden and design the garden surrounding it
d: finish going through the cupboards in the house and clearing out.

Now you know what you want, and hopefully you have made a list for each of the areas, this book will help you determine what you need to do to achieve these goals.

Chapter 5
Differentiating between internal and external pain

You have now got your mind to think in a whole new way, so I will continue to share my story of how I got to all these answers.

In 2000 I was on the ever present hunt for someone to help me get over my pain from the accident. I had already been to every physio I knew of, or at each course I would get the physio offering the course to evaluate me and provide some insight and then go and see them for some treatment sessions. I had tried Pilates, mobilization, Reiki healing and crystal therapy. I even went to a chiropractor and he manipulated my spine and gave me injections. After the second treatment I was admitted into hospital with kidney stones, this was 5 years after my accident. My kidney stones seem to occur every 10 years with other physical misfortunes in between.

When I did my time line, I was stunned to notice that my major events seemed to occur every 5 years in the beginning. It seems to have sped up with more frequent events later on, which I think was a way to force me into making a stand and analyzing why I am like I am and why these things happen to me. Well this was 2000. I woke up that morning with severe pain in my side and feeling very nauseous. I was having cold sweats and really didn't feel well as I had severe pain in my side. I drove myself to the doctor early that morning before work, after testing my urine for blood in it, they informed me that I had a kidney stone and gave me some medication to relax the urethra. He told me to drink lots of water and that I would pass the stone and then I would be fine. I worked an entire day with fever sweats and pain in my side assuming the stone would pass.

It feels like a shark is biting you in your side. I was nauseous and really didn't feel good. During the second last patient I had to apologize profusely and take myself to the hospital as I could no longer stand the pain. It gets a bit ridiculous when you are sitting with your head resting on their head while you are trying to massage their neck and back, suffering in silence and zoning out when the pain grabs you and the fever sweat comes.

When you get admitted for kidney stones they always try to get you to pass them naturally by pumping you full of saline. My body seems to be stubborn and refuses to let the stones go naturally so they had to operate the next morning to remove them. Technology has improved so drastically that they scope up your bladder and either crush the stone or zap it with a laser. When they do this, they put a stent in (straw with a string) to prevent your urethra from swelling shut. This you have to keep in for 2 weeks and then they remove it again. Luckily it has a little string, much like a tampon, so you can just pull it out after the swelling has come down two weeks after the surgery.

I am grateful that they don't have to remove the kidney stone like they did in the olden days. I have seen a number of patients who have massive scars over their ribs from kidney stones being removed in the past. That must have been really sore. Imagine doing that 4 times or more!!! One would be man down a lot longer than 2 weeks.

I was back at work the day after I was discharged, why I do this is beyond me. I suppose our mentality is no work, no pay, as I was working as a locum during that time. Or it's the fact that I can't let people down. Even now working for myself I have no work, no pay, but I do have insurance to help when I am booked off. I still work when I shouldn't and it's this guilt feeling of not being able to help those that need more help than me. I know what's wrong with me and I can get better.

So two weeks later I went dressed in my hockey gear, ready to have my stent removed before the game. The sisters were preparing me for a full anaesthetic, when I was under the impression that it was going to be a local, as I had a game in 2 hours, much to their horror. Also they could not do full anaesthetic as I had eaten breakfast. So I asked them to phone the Doctor and ask him if he could do it under local. The doctor did do it under local. Apparently the only reason why he does it under general is to remove the mental discomfort the patient would experience while he is grovelling down at your privates.

So I had the local and was out in a few minutes as opposed to longer, so I could go and play hockey. I did play my game, but I really should have rested, as in hindsight I was not at my best health and did not enjoy it as much as I could have. I remember the game, it was a memory imprinted in my brain and better than just going through the motions of everyday life with no memories that stick out.

A few months down the line I had another kidney stone on the other side and had to go through the whole process again. At this stage I already knew the drill and they just removed the stent in his rooms, which was much easier and cheaper. I must say the Doctor thought I was mad when I told him that I had a kidney stone before he had even done any tests. He looked at me and said: "How do you know?" I told him that I had had it before and knew the feeling.

Kidney stone pain is not a pain you forget and is worse than labour pains. At least with labour pains, you don't feel nauseous, and you don't get fever sweats and you get a present when you are finished dying. You also get a respite between contractions, not so with kidney stones. With kidney stones you are permanently nauseous and feel your whole body goosing with pain and fever. You have excruciating pain that doubles you over and you are not able to walk up straight. There is no position that is even remotely comfortable, so you constantly fidget and the fidgeting just makes the pain worse. The morphine or Pethadine gives you a wonderful respite, but when it wears off you are back to hell.

I remember my first experience with Pethadine. As they injected it, I could feel it moving through my body from my right arm to my left arm and then down my legs. I felt light and not quite with it and had lost all spatial orientation. My dad said I walked like a buffalo; I looked bizarre and was walking with my legs exaggerated while stepping forward and not knowing where they were when I put them down. My arms were outstretched trying to gain my balance and it was slow and hilarious.

Soon after my kidney stones episode I moved to the UK to work. Here I continued to try different Physios to decrease my pains. It was here that I drank the Chinese concoction that didn't work.

At this stage my pain was not really under control. I was still getting severe cramping over my ribs on my back and dead legs if I sat for too long. Coccyx pain if I sat on a hard chair. It literally felt like my coccyx was breaking off. I was convinced of this and have had many patients since then tell me the same story. However, your coccyx is 2 cm away from the chair, so it's not the coccyx but actually your gluteus maximus trigger point you are sitting on which refers pain to the coccyx. Get rid of the trigger point and you get rid of the coccyx pain. I used to get cramping of my muscles and increased pain if I cycled too often. So I cycled to work on a Monday and left my bike there for the week and cycled back on Friday. It was only a 15 minute cycle, which is really not that far, but all I could manage.

It was 10 years after my first kidney stones that I got my third kidney stone and again both sides were blocked. They were blocked so badly that the 5 bags of saline they pumped through me did not come out the other side. Again I felt the pain of the shark biting me in my side, combined with nausea and fever and I knew it was the kidney stones talking again. I went to the hospital and confirmed my theory with the tests they do.

As it was on a Sunday my medical aid was not available and thus no authorization was provided, but we went ahead as both kidneys were blocked and you cannot leave that as you can die. They operated early the next morning as the 5 bags of saline they pumped through had not rinsed the stones out. However this time round when I woke from the anaesthetic, I was struggling to breathe. My saturation was good, but it felt as if I could not expand my lungs enough to get air in and I kept asking the nurses to sit me up right instead of giving me oxygen, which made me more anxious.

Of course by the time I got to the room, I knew the drill was that I must pee before I was discharged. So I hauled myself out of bed and then peed and got ready to leave. By the time I got home, I was not feeling well. I was struggling to breathe and could not lie flat on the bed as I could not breathe. I could not even walk around the bed as I was out of breath. My legs and arms were swollen and I was wondering if I had an embolism from the anaesthetic. I called my dad, who is a doctor, who told me to go back to the hospital.

When I arrived back at the hospital at the emergency room, I told the nurses there that I had been operated on that morning by the urologist and that they must please call him. They insisted that they continue to do the work up before they call the Doctor. They gave me a cup to pee in and when it came back just with blood, they assumed I was menstruating even though I kept telling them that I had surgery that morning. Maybe I didn’t speak clearly as I was struggling to breathe. They continued to do the work up and then discharged me stating there was nothing wrong with me. I felt rather frustrated and worried.

A few days later the Doctor called me to ask what was going on as no one had called him when I was in the emergency room. He checked on me and it was decided that I may have a slight allergic reaction to the anaesthetic. In my opinion, I think it was the fact that I had 5 bags of saline pumped into me and didn't pee once. So the fluid had to go somewhere other than out. This made me swollen everywhere, my ankles, my fingers and around my lungs as the fluid just moves in to all the cells. Unfortunately when you have both kidneys involved at the same time, it means nothing is working properly. It also means that they can't operate on both sides at the same time, as there can be too much swelling and cause further damage, so I had the other kidney stone removed 6 weeks later.

While I was recovering, I had to fight with the medical aid, as they were refusing to pay my medical bills because it was not a hospital they support. As I am in the industry I know all the terminology they use and what they will and won't pay for. This was very useful as it was an emergency PMB condition (prescribed minimum benefit) and if I didn't get the operation I would have died. When they hear this terminology they didn't even bat an eye and just paid everything. With a bit of perseverance I was able to resolve all the issues and was able to continue with the second procedure 6 weeks later.

This little episode of my kidney stone caused me to be bed ridden for two weeks, before I felt well enough to see my patients. In hind sight I think I should have taken a bit more time off. Another week might have been better.

When it was time to do the second kidney stone the doctor informed me that I would have to stay overnight to ensure nothing happened. I reluctantly agreed. I had a seminar taking place on the weekend, and I had scheduled my surgery to take place on the Thursday, thinking it would not be that bad as it was not sore like the others were when I had emergency surgery. My husband refused to let me go to the seminar on the Friday night, as he said that he thought I was mad. So I went on the Saturday. After the first 3 hours session, I was feeling very sorry for myself, thinking that I should go home. But there is something in me that if I have paid for a course, come hell or high water, I am going to go as I am not going to lose my money just because I didn't feel well. So I was sitting on the grass feeling very sorry for myself, when another lady sat down beside me and asked me what was wrong.

I told her I had just had kidney surgery and had no pain pills on me and was dying of the pain and feeling very grim. She informed me that she actually worked in the kidney department, taking the scans of the kidneys to determine the stones and that she had some marvellous pain meds on her and gave me some. She was my hero for the day. I managed to feel good enough to last through till the end of the session which lasted till late that night and I attended the Sunday session. I don't think I took time off work with this kidney stone but again I think a week would have gone down well in hind sight.

I remember my little boy being worried about me. He would lie in bed next to me and set up all the kids' movies on the laptop. They are really amazing and learn how to use the equipment so fast. He was only 3 years old and his motto was "If you are sick, you must stay in bed and watch DVDs and push pause to go vomit". Love it. He also made me food, where he would bring me an apple and make toast and then he would try and feed me while I was sleeping. Bless his little heart. I truly think he would make a wonderful caring Doctor one day, if this is what he chooses to do.

So now I know what the kidney stones feel like and when I feel my kidneys twitching in my body and feel a little bit of discomfort. I make sure I increase my water intake and sometimes I take some citric soda. The problem though with kidneys that don't work properly, is that they can cause your feet to swell on those really hot days. Also they tend to swell when you fly.

I remember when we flew to New York, by the time we landed there, my feet and even my legs were so swollen, that I was really uncomfortable. It made walking those long blocks in New York very difficult and by the time we reached the park I had had enough walking and only wanted to go back to the house where we were staying. A few of my patients have the same misfortune of swelling in their legs on those hot days. The one lady in particular has such bad swelling in her legs that her legs have gone hard and feel literally like bone instead of soft and pliable. By improving her kidney function and adding some special supplementation from good neutraceutical companies to help the kidneys, she has soft, pliable legs now and the pains she was experiencing in her legs have reduced significantly.

What I have learnt though is the importance of eating healthy and drinking lots of water, as I never used to drink a lot of water or any other beverage for that matter. You need to drink at least 0.033 x body weight in Kg, to ensure you are getting enough water through your system. Kidney stones are not something I want to experience again and drinking water helps to prevent this.

Chapter 6
The whiplash

At this stage I was still in full swing on learning about pain and suffering in my personal life. I had not recovered from my car accident yet and still experienced severe cramping throughout my body. I had only had the two kidney stones, so was still not drinking much water. I was trying to do some sport in the form of cycling. I was working in the UK and had been there since 2001. Of course there you are able to cycle to work and back or catch the bus, not like in South Africa where it is either too far or you will be killed by the Taxis or hijacked by someone off the streets.

It was 2005 and I was cycling to work on the Monday when I was knocked off my bike: a car had clipped my back tire. I had my helmet on and a backpack on my back. I fell on my back hitting my head so hard on the tar that my helmet cracked. I was stunned for a few seconds before I got up and analysed my body, didn't seem too bad apart from the swelling that was taking place on my shin. I was too sore to get back on my bike and ride the last little block to work, so I walked to work and showered and continued through my day.

As the day progressed my neck got progressively stiffer and stiffer on the front and I had pain over my left front rib cage. I also had a massive hematoma on my shin. But I continued with my work and even gave a Pilates class that evening. I was unable to kneel on my right knee and kept having to tell the class that they must put their knees down as they were following what I was doing and not what I was saying. Classic example of do what I say and not what I do. So I then had to kneel on the sore leg so they could just follow what they were supposed to be doing.

I never went for treatment or even X-rays, but I had a whiplash injury of my neck. This is what I do, for my work is to analyse people who have been in accidents and determine their injuries. My neck was very stiff and sore. So as I advise all my patients to do, I started stretching it side to side and to the front and put heat on it. I got full range back quite soon, but I still had muscle spasm of my sternocleidomastoid muscle, which causes dizziness and headaches. I was unable to lie on my left side due to my injury to the stomach muscle. My abdominal muscle on the left where it attaches onto the ribs had been torn and it now still cramps from time to time and is rather a nuisance. As this muscle was torn, and its action is to help keep the ribs in position, I now have a rib that clicks when I lie on my left side as the rib shifts out of position.

The only thing that got better with some treatment was the hematoma, but even that took a while to get better. Sometimes a hematoma can leave a large lump where it was. One needs to put ice on the hematoma for the first 3 days and massage the lump down after a few weeks changing to heat over the hematoma. You keep moving the big lump from side to side breaking it up, so that the body can reabsorb it, eventually it will return to normal.

Now the pains got ridiculous. When my back cramped, I would hunch my back like the hunchback of Notre dame, this then resulted in my stomach cramping on my left lower ribs. So I then twisted my back backwards. It was a sight to see. I learnt very quickly that I cannot allow my body to get cold at all. The UK is much colder than South Africa but their houses and work places are really well equipped with heating indoors, so it's the change from indoors to outdoors that can make your body cramp if not well dressed. I would make sure I had long-jons on and every inch of my body was covered well so as not to get cold at all. It is all about the layers. This has been a good thing to know as it has helped a lot with my pain. I will no longer look fashionable just for the sake of fashion, if it makes me get cold. Or you make sure your jerseys are both fashionable and warm.

I started getting heart palpitations when I exercised or for no apparent reason and my sinuses were so badly blocked that I would snore myself awake and suffer with dry cracked lips permanently. If I went for an afternoon nap, my eyelids would swell shut. I went for regular treatment but could not understand why the treatment I was getting was not helping. Everything was getting worse and nothing was helping. Some days I would cry from pain and frustration especially if the body got cold, or when I was cycling home and my body was complaining and I could not stop as I was not on the bus route. It only took me 15-20 minutes to cycle home, but it felt like a life-time, it was quicker than the bus and I was determined to try some form of exercise to try and get my body better. If my legs weren't cramping then it felt like my coccyx was breaking off and my buttocks went numb and then my legs went numb and my arms would pull and I was uncomfortable everywhere. All the muscles were stiff and sore and had orange peel in my arms and my legs and my back. I had orange peel everywhere, making my skin tight everywhere.

It was during this time that I got introduced to a technique called IMS (intramuscular stimulation). I do not believe in going out to look for courses. If I am interested in a course, I will think about what course I would like to do, and when someone mentions a course to me that I am interested in I will go on it. If I don't hear about the course then it's not meant to be. So I was working in St Helliers' hospital in the UK and there was another South African who was really interested in attending the IMS course which was taking place that weekend in London. However, she was unable to go as she was flying back home on the Friday night. I took the details and called them and went. This course changed the way I treated patients forever.

Professor Chan Gunn who comes from Canada, who invented the words radiculopathy and neuropathy was teaching this course. He is a little man who took me up to my shoulder, but he is brilliant. He has studied so many different things and has a pain clinic in Canada implementing these techniques. He is the most amazing person to listen to. I hung on his every word. He told us that you must treat the whole body not just the area of pain. He said that if you have a problem with the muscle, that it will cause a problem in the tendon. But if you release the muscle, you will release the tendon too. He said that if you do not respond to IMS that the problem is not muscular but metabolic. This means that it was crucial to look at the person's diet and supplementation program, or you will never get them better.

He showed us what the normal range of motion was for every joint. He said that you must check all the joints and ensure that when you are working on the person that you work to getting full range of the body in each joint, just to fix the one area. When the body can move freely, then the person will have no pain. He mentioned that the body has clues to indicate where the problems are and showed us how to see these clues. One of them was the orange peel. Many people call orange peel cellulite and think that it is because they are fat. However, orange peel is an indication that the muscle is tight below the orange peel and if you release the muscle you will get soft pliable skin with no orange peel. Your skin should pick up like puppy dog skin everywhere on the body. If it does not, then you release the body until it does.

This reminds me of a story I often tell to my patients to explain this point. I was newly qualified and had been treating a man for headaches and sore neck on his right side. After the third unsuccessful treatment I noticed he was limping and I asked him what was wrong with his foot. He said nothing. I asked then why he was limping, he mentioned that 15 years prior, he had torn his calf muscle and had surgery to fix it. I asked if he had ever had treatment afterwards for the calf and he said that he had not. He did not have full range of his ankle and could barely get 90 degrees flexion. So I suggested he did a calf stretch every 2 hours until he had full range of movement.

At the next session as he was waiting for me to finish the patient before him, he was stretching his calf out. He said that he had set his alarm for every two hours, as recommended, and as he worked in a warehouse and was a manager of quite a few people, he would make every one stop and stretch their legs out. Within four days he had full range of movement of his ankle and he also reported that the pain he had under his foot since the surgery had gone and so had his neck pain.

Gunn's theories really made sense and spoke to my way of thinking. He showed us so many ways of seeing the problems without even talking to the patient. These theories helped me treat patients with trigger fingers, back to full range without surgery, as it is about releasing the muscle in the forearm which is making the tendon in the fingers tight and stuck. I remember having a patient who had claw hand, never mind trigger finger. I focused on releasing his entire forearm, both front and back. It only took me 4 sessions with the needles to get rid of his claw hand and both he and I were ecstatic.

Working at the government hospital was really great. I was head of the department there and I had a number of Physio's and Physio students and assistants under my supervision. I learnt a lot about management and writing of reports and discharge reports and basic good communication between your colleagues. We constantly had students who had to shadow us for 4-6 weeks. I would always get the patient to tell the student when they were pushing as hard as I was, so that they know how hard they should be working on their patients. Many of the students' eyes nearly popped out when they finally got the right pressure. The secret is in using your body weight. Also the pressure must be effective. It is going to be sore, but must never be that sore that you want to get off the bed.

I had another patient who would lie on the bed and cry, "eina! eina! (ouch, Ouch), that is so nice!" then you know you have it just right or if they get goose bumps when you are working on them. At the time of the Gunn course, I had a student who was constantly raving about this nutrition course his brother had attended. I had not really been paying much attention as it was not something I thought I was interested in, but after the course when Gunn himself said that you need to look at nutrition, I asked this guy to give me the details of the course.

As it so happened the course was literally a week or two later and not too far either, so I booked and arranged accommodation and went on the "Nutrition and lifestyle course – by Paul Check"

He is a gentleman who has been studying nutrition and exercise for a number of years and based his information on the book by William Wolcott "The metabolic typing diet". I remember the course as if it was yesterday as my problems had been progressively getting worse and not responding to any form of treatment and now I knew why. During Paul's course we had to complete the HAQ and then he would discuss each aspect in detail as to why it was like that and that diet and supplementation was the key.

So this course came in the nick of time. I had thought that I was eating healthily and did not realize that food can have such a huge impact on ones' health. I used to eat pizza every Friday night without fail. I would eat sweets regularly, some mornings waking up and eating fruit pastels that were lying on my bedside table, because I could. There is nothing nicer than the buy one, get one free promotions they have in the UK, so I would eat Lasagne every night and with that I would eat a tin of corn. I would also buy either a cheese cake or Pavlova or lemon meringue each week and consume it all by myself. It was lovely, but also very unhealthy. It took me a year to realize that I was getting diarrhoea from eating the pizza and when I discovered this I stopped eating it immediately, even though it was on my cheat day.

Within two weeks of eating correctly according to my results from the book, I had cleared my sinuses. Most of my complaints started to go away, like the sinus and the swollen eye. I started losing the weight I had gained. I learnt a lot on this course and was able to help many people afterwards. There was this one lady who had been to a Dietician and she was eating everything right. The only mistake that she made is that after each evening meal she would have a slice of apple pie. Now I understood her vice very clearly, but I also know now that you can't have sugar and sweets and all things nice every day. I limit it to Fridays now. My son even calls it junk day. So for the entire week I eat correctly and drink my water and do everything right, then on Friday I get pizza and eat a sweet and watch a movie. Then we climb back on the wagon again. According to Paul, out of 21 meals for the week, you may cheat 3 of them. I would add that this is if you are already healthy. If you are sick you need to keep on the straight and narrow wagon until your symptoms are gone. If this is too difficult then cheat, but know that your body is taking strain and that it is difficult to stay on the wagon if you constantly cheat.

At the course I learnt about the 6 fundamental factors of being healthy and took them to heart. On my return to SA I would teach these factors to my patients and I actually set up a course teaching Physios about these factors too. The factors will be discussed in detail later in the book, but for now they are, thoughts, breathing, water intake, food/vitamin intake, exercise and sleep. You need to have a balance of all the areas to be healthy in mind and body. It is not easy to do, but once you start and get going, it is easy to maintain once you know what to do and once you are in a routine.

I had spent 4 years in the UK on an extreme upward curve to educate myself, so that I could get myself better and then I used the knowledge I gained at the different courses to treat my patients and see what worked and what didn't work. It was an amazing journey and still is.

We returned to South Africa and I opened my chronic pain practice. When I was working in the UK, because the waiting list is so long to see a physio, either your injury has fixed itself or you now have chronic pain. The waiting list there is between 4-6months to see a person for treatment. Then you are only allowed to have 6 treatments, after which you get discharged. Most of the Physios get taught that you must only give exercises as if you touch the patient, they will become dependent on you and you will never be able to get rid of them.

What I learnt from the people in the UK is that when you give them an exercise to do, that they will do it till the day they die, all to help themselves. When I asked them to do the stretch every two hours, they would ask if they should do it at night, thus wake up from sleep, which is how seriously they take the advice given to them. I spent a lot of time teaching the Physios there about trigger points, as it was not part of their education and many of them didn't even know what it is. Trigger points have been a huge part of my life and my education and I have even set up a course to initially teach the UK Physios I worked with, in a course form and then later advanced the course to teach the South African Physios.

I was known in the UK as the physio to send the complicated patients to. The senior twos and junior Physios who were under my supervision would always come and ask for advice and if they felt it was above their means, they would refer the patient to my care. I ignored the 6 session rule, as there is no way you can get a patient better in 6 sessions if they have chronic pain. It takes months. So I would see them for about 4-6 sessions over a four week period, then they would be given a ton of advice to do and I would monitor them on a monthly basis until they could continue on their own. They managed wonderfully. Many patients who had suffered for a long time were pain free. What I did learn though is that not everyone and I am case in point, can exercise the pain away. Sometimes exercise makes the problem worse, but there is a fine line too of when you do need to go back to exercising.

I had a patient who had fallen off his horse and hurt his left shoulder. He was unable to lift the arm and experienced severe pain down the arm. I treated him a few sessions and his pain was improving significantly, but he was too scared to ride his horse again. His arm seemed to not want to get the last bit of strength back and was not responding to further treatment. It came to a point where I told him that he needs to get back on the horse to get the final strength back and thus get rid of the last bit of pain. He did so with hesitation, but reported back to me that it had been a huge success and that he was feeling amazing.

There was another patient who had been operated on for a knee replacement and was refusing to walk as his leg was too painful. The other Physios were telling me that he was just full of it and too lazy to get going. In actual fact the problem was that he had a huge trigger point in his leg which was causing such severe pain that he physically was not able to lift the leg and it felt very weak. I released the trigger point and he got up and walked. Here exercise would have made the problem worse, but once the trigger point was released, exercise is good to do again.

So when your body has been injured such as mine and it does not respond to treatment, such as mine, you need to do a combination of things to get it better. Only doing one thing such as only doing treatment or only taking medication is not going to fix the problem. You need to get regular treatment with needles. Then you need to focus on eating correctly and making sure you take the correct supplements to ensure you correct the vitamin deficiencies. Once you start feeling better you can add a light exercise regime in and then gradually build it up to the level you want to take it to. The key is to find the right people to motivate you to go through the different stages and to help you along the way.

My whiplash did have lingering lasting effects. From time to time the muscle in my neck will complain and cause dizziness and it sometimes is affected by driving on circle onramps. If one turns your head fast you feel dizzy or if you go to lie down in your bed then the room spins. This is all due to the muscle in the front of your neck. It is also responsible for causing nausea, tearing of your eye and severe headaches on your forehead. This muscle is often missed by people as they always tend to focus on the back of your neck, but you will feel that the ropes on the front of your neck are tight and sore, then you can massage it yourself to ease the pain.

Many of my patients who have had whiplash injuries, have this muscle activated and they suffer for many years with dizziness and headaches. A few sessions of needles and massage and the problem is brought under control and if it does get problematic, you will know exactly what to do to help yourself.

With chronic pain the most important thing is knowledge. As said in the book "The greatness in you" by Seanaphoka Tapi. *"There is no wealth more rewarding than education and information. Seek it and it will enlighten and liberate you forever."*

Chapter 7
The pregnancy and incontinence

It was 2006 and I was back in South Africa working with some other Physios specializing in chronic pain. I was only back a few months when I found out I was pregnant. This was a challenge on my body, as it had been pain free for 2 years after attending the IMS sessions with a Physio in England. I was at the peak of my health, eating correctly and sleeping correctly and feeling amazing. The change in my body shape caused all my spasms to return, luckily not to the extent of before, but bad enough that I was desperate for the needles.

I remember the one day having a severe headache, which I was not allowed to take any pills for. I was begging the Physios to put a needle in my neck to release the headaches. They refused stating they were too scared in case I lost the baby. I kept telling them that considering I was a dry needle addict and that I was not scared of the needles, that it would be fine. They still refused. So I needled myself. The areas I could reach got zapped and those that couldn't be reached I got my mother to needle for me. It was heaven on earth, as my headache instantly went away. This is how powerful a needle can be. Way better than taking a tablet that just eases the pain for the time being, but when it wears off, it's back again.

The other thing that I discovered was how great swimming is when you are pregnant. It is the most amazing feeling, as you really don't feel like you are pregnant. I remember the one afternoon being so hot and sore that I decided I would go and swim. When I got in, I felt the weight lift off my body and suddenly my back pain was gone; it was wonderful and super refreshing.

During my early pregnancy I was treating a lady who had been bed ridden for two years because of a pain she was experiencing in her ischial tuberosity where the hamstring inserts. The pain was so bad that she was unable to stand or sit and could only lie down, even rolling over caused severe pain in her buttock area.

I treated her over a space of a few months. On evaluation I found she had severe gluteal muscle spasm as well as hamstring muscle spasm. She was complaining of back pain and leg pain and it had all started when she went walking on a treadmill with weights on her legs. Although I eased the secondary pain as a result of the initial problem, I could never find the source of her pain. A few months later, I myself experienced the same pain. I was about 6 months pregnant when I started to feel severe pain on my right ischial tuberosity (sit Bone), just on the inside of the bone. We call it the medial part of your ischial tuberosity. This is where your hamstring inserts, which is why I focused on her hamstring and gluteal area. It is also where the pelvic floor inserts on the inner side. So when I found I was having trouble turning at night and found it painful to sit on, I started hunting it down. I finally tracked it down to my pelvic floor muscle and came to the conclusion that it was because of my sons head pushing on my pelvic floor. I called her immediately and asked her to come in to check. Within three treatments, we had resolved the problem.

To find said problem one needs to evaluate the pelvic floor inserting your fingers into your vagina, just inside. You then visualize the area like a clock and check one o'clock, two o'clock etc. feeling for little tight bits that feel like dental floss, but are sore to touch. You then press the area until the pain goes away and your problem is resolved. Other techniques that can be used are Shortwave and a pelvic floor stimulator.

It was also brought to my attention that there are many people who have pelvic floor problems who experience pain with menstruation or pain with intercourse. These muscles are activated through a range of causes such as chronic on-going pain throughout the body. Any injury to the area can cause this problem, like a tear in the pelvic floor during the birthing process or a fall on the coccyx.

This doesn't just happen in women; men can also have this problem. One of the other tools I use to help alleviate this problem, is to place a vaginal probe inside the vagina and then send a TENS current through it, very nice and relaxing. For men we would use an anal probe. This same probe can also be used to improve incontinence as this is caused again due to an injury to this muscle causing spasm and pain which then results in incontinence, the current is slightly different.

Although I had experienced pain on my ischial tuberosity, it was about to get a lot worse. My pregnancy was uncomplicated, but because I felt I was not ready and had a few more things to do before I could deliver, I suppressed my birth for about 5 days. I went into labour the Thursday morning. I had arranged that a Doula would help me during my birthing process as she would be able to tell me when I needed to go to the hospital or if I was still okay at home. So when I called her she said she would come through and help me through the day. As soon as she arrived, my contractions wilted away, so she left later in the day. The next morning the same thing happened and when she came through the contractions stopped.

She came through about 4 times. Finally on Tuesday she said to me that we needed to do a workshop on facing the tiger. Basically analyse why you are suppressing the birthing process and conquer your fears. We did this and I went out to the farm to visit my cat, all part of the process. At about midday, she then went home. At 4 o'clock that afternoon I went into labour again and the contractions were very strong. When I called her I asked her to wait before she came, to make sure the contractions were not going to stop again. After about an hour I called her again to tell her that she must come as they were very strong. She spent the evening rubbing my back and adding pressure over the sacrum when the contractions came. She also timed the contractions and at 3 in the morning she said we were ready to go to the hospital. When I got there, because I had been experiencing stress over the past week, they decided to break my water to make sure baby was okay. By 5am on the Wednesday morning I had my little baby boy. I had delivered him in a water birth, which was amazing. The water definitely helps in reducing pain and created a wonderful atmosphere that felt we weren't even in the hospital.

One thing I can say is that when you are pushing that massive head out, do not help your vaginal wall by pulling it more. I had done this on the right side, which resulted in me tearing my vagina quite badly on the inside. This did not get picked up and thus I did not get stitches. I kept wondering why my right side of my vagina was so painful and that I could not sit properly for weeks. I had to put ice on it for a long time. At my 6 week check-up, the Gynae informed me that I had torn it quite badly and that it had now formed a scar. This was also the reason why at 4 weeks after the birth, when I decided that I wanted to do 30min of weeding, sitting on my haunches pulling out little weeds, that I became incontinent.

We are taught at university, that recovery from birth takes about 6 weeks for your body to get marginally get back to normal, but only 3 years before your hormones return to normal. So no heavy exercise is to be done in the first 6 weeks while your body is readjusting to normal. This is basically for any injury. It takes 3 days inflammation, then on day four your body starts to repair the damage. By day 21 (3 weeks) most of the repair has been done and gentle stretching can be done to get full range with light balance or reeducation exercises to be done. At 6 weeks you can return to normal exercise regimes, building the strength up gradually till you are back to your original regime. Sometimes this can take up to 6 months before you are allowed to use heavy weights to exercise with.

But at 4 weeks I felt wonderful. My baby was eating every 6 hours which was heaven. He slept in between all the time. He was a really easy baby. I kept thinking that one should go back to work immediately and then take off 3 months when they get a bit bigger and sleep less. The problem with me weeding for the 30 min, was not the fact that weeding is really easy to do, it was the fact that sitting on my haunches increases abdominal pressure intensely and this pressure on the pelvic floor which had been torn, resulted in me being stress incontinent for 2 years.

There are two types of incontinence, stress and urge incontinent. Stress incontinence means that when you cough or sneeze especially when your bladder is full, you are guaranteed to pee down your leg. Urge incontinence is when your bladder is full and you are on your way to the toilet, that you physically just can't keep it in, so once again you pee yourself. Both are awful.

To improve pelvic floor strength you will need those pelvic floor applicators that I mentioned before which are inserted like a tampon. You then attach it to a pelvic floor stimulating machine that sends impulses to your muscles to help them contract. You attach this machine to your belt and continue to do your things around the house. It is a bit uncomfortable to sit with this, so either you lie and read a book for the 30min while its working your pelvic floor, or you go for a walk. I found it most bazar how after my injury I was unable to feel my pelvic floor contract on the right, even though I had been teaching it for years to my patients. But it was because I had damaged the muscle itself and it was so weak that I could not feel it contracting. The other problem I experienced after the birth, when I started menstruating again, was severe pain on my ischial tuberosity. This time it was both sides. I felt I needed to walk around holding my bottom on my ischial bones just to ease the pain, but this did nothing. I just looked funny.

I sat on hot bean bags, which did help to an extent, but I would not understand why my sit bones felt like they wanted to fall off during my menstrual cycle. I am sure many of you have felt that your fanny wants to fall off during menstruation, I have had that before, myself, but this was different area totally. When I mentioned this to my Gynae she palmed it off saying it was my SI joint. This was definitely not my SI joint. So I hit the books and found that at the bottom of your pelvis you have a triangle muscle that runs from the ischial tuberosity on the right to the ischial tuberosity on the left and then form the both sides to the coccyx, making a little triangle that the baby comes through. This is the bottom of your pelvic floor, and I suspect the one I injured during the birthing process. So I had shortening of the right sided one, which if you remember from the Chan Gunn information, my entire area was pulled out of balance. When you menstruate, you have increased pressure pushing on these muscles and that activates the trigger point causing the pain. Once again a bit of heat and the pelvic floor stimulator and I used the shortwave machine I have at my disposal to treat the area and it came right.

Thank goodness I no longer have the pain anymore and only from time to time when I am not feeling well does my pelvic floor play up and I want to pee myself.

I now make it part of my general treatment to ask if my ladies have problems with menstruating or pain with intercourse as it can easily be resolved with a plug in a special place while I am working on the other areas, a two in one combo. I often think that it is such an uncomfortable topic to talk about to the doctor and most of them just say that it is normal so they must just take pain pills. But you should not really experience pain when you menstruate. Perhaps when you first start as its weird and your body needs to adjust, but it should never been that painful.

Many women have also commented that they became incontinent after a hysterectomy. My theory is that the pelvic floor got hurt during the procedure and this would cause the pain from the muscle spasms that were created. Also by improving your pelvic floor strength, you will be able to support your bladder as well as your vagina and could potentially prevent them from prolapsing. So ladies get the pelvic floor strengthened up! There are many ways of doing this. First you need to contract the muscle. If you don't know where it is tighten your anus only, when you do this you should feel it tightening in the vagina area too. For the men, they must focus on pulling up their balls while sitting. If you have stress incontinence, so you pee when you cough or sneeze, then you need to be able to contract your muscles fast. So you need to tighten, relax and tighten and relax over and over aiming to do 100. If you are urge incontinence, pee when your bladder is full. You need to hold the pelvic floor tight for 10 counts and relax and repeat it 50 times. You can make a habit of doing it when brushing your teeth, or when you are driving to work and stop at the traffic lights. But you need to do it often to get results.

Secondly, you can purchase a pelvic floor stimulator machine, which you then use on a daily basis to improve the strength by going for a walk or lying on your bed reading while having this working on your muscles. This is by far the best method. You can also combine the exercise using the machine as you will be able to feel precisely where you need to be tightening your muscles.

Focus on getting healthier in your body and mind, by doing the other things mentioned in this book. It is very important to stay as active as you can for as long as you can and to work as long as you can to keep your mind active and young. Work is not necessarily physically going to work, but rather to keep busy with tasks at home and making new goals to achieve each year. Not sitting on the couch watching TV all day, which is not good for your body at all. I saw a picture of two ladies who were both in their 70s. The one was old and frail and sitting in a chair with her walking frame and the other looked like she was in her thirties. She was well defined and muscles rippling everywhere. Which one do you want to look like?

Chapter 8
The pivotal point of information through adrenal fatigue

Time has been ticking on and I have by now had the car accident, 4 kidney stone episodes, the whiplash injury and the incontinence issues. I am gatvol (fed-up) of getting injured, but have my pains pretty much under control in that I know how to treat them when they get bothersome. It took me 10 years to find someone who could needle my body and release most of the areas of pain enough that I could manage it from there and enable me to follow the diet and other lifestyle changes. I know how far I can push myself and am ready to take on a new challenge of Belly dancing as my form of exercise to get fit and supple. It is gentle enough that I do not get headaches and other pains, but intense enough that my muscles would cramp for the first year over my thoracic area where I broke my ribs. Fortunately I know that adding pressure using the corner of the wall over the muscle in spasm, eases it up, so half the class I spent leaning up against the wall and the other half of the class I spent getting the area moving.

It was 2012 and I was chatting to a friend who was unable to have kids. She mentioned that her eggs did not mature properly and because she was getting older, almost 40, she didn't have much time to have her own child and that she and her husband were thinking of using a donor egg. I was telling her that she must be careful of who's eggs she chose as even though the medical history was good, you never know what the person's personality is like or what they like or dislike or how clever they are or how they express themselves. Before I knew it I told her she should have mine. Now once I make a promise to someone, I do not go back on my word.

So I was tied by my honour. We started the process and by the end of 2012 we harvested my first eggs.

If I had even thought about this a bit better or investigated it a bit more, I think I would have said no. In hindsight I will advise anyone thinking of doing this that it could potentially be the biggest mistake of their lives. The story ahead has been the most difficult experience I have had to go through, and not the harvesting, but the effects the harvesting had on the body after it was done.

When harvesting eggs, you have to get your menstrual cycles to sync with the mom to be. This gets done by putting you on the same hormone pill to make you start menstruating on the same day. When you are in sink you then start injecting special hormones every day at the exact same time to stimulate the ovaries to produce more eggs. The time issue is a big factor of this whole procedure and you have to within 30min of the previous day's injection make sure you inject again. Once the eggs are 2cm large, which is determined by sonar on a regular basis, they are harvested under light anaesthetic (dormicum) in a special procedure room.

A week before the first harvesting I was attending a course when I suddenly experienced blurred vision and my pupils were pin point size. It felt like I was having an aura just before you have a migraine, but no headache came on and no nausea. I could not see any writing on the board and felt very funny. Not funny ha ha, but funny not good. Disorientated because I couldn't see and waiting for the headache to come one. When I called the neurologist I work with, he asked if I was taking any hormone therapy and told me that I was having a hormonal migraine. This was quite a relief as I was wondering if I was having a stroke. I must say if I had realized that the hormonal migraines were going to continue for years after the event I would not have continued. Doing the injections and putting such high dosages of hormones in my body disrupted the hormonal balance. This does not right itself either.

So I continued and I remember the night before my first harvest, I had to inject a hormone at a very specific time so that my eggs were released at a very specific time the next morning so that the Doctor could organize his day and harvest me at that exact time when the eggs were released. How I remember this is that our belly dancing school was performing a concert that same night. I remember my stomach feeling very uncomfortable, what with 9 eggs each measuring 2cm in diameter being shaken around. So between the dances when we had to change our costumes, I had to whip out the injection, mix the meds and jab the tummy in a cloakroom full of people all watching and asking what on earth was going on. I danced my heart out with my tummy draping lavishly over my belly belt and the next day I went in for the procedure. By the time I got home only a few hours after the procedure, I was up and about. I did feel a bit uncomfortable especially on the left side, but carried on as normal.

The nine eggs that were harvested gave her three opportunities as they insert 2-3 eggs in at a time. As soon as they have harvested the eggs they insert the newly acquired sperm and then monitor the eggs to see if they become fertilized. This takes about a week. Once this has occurred they then insert the actively growing cells into the uterus and hope they implant. She had three tries using these eggs, but unfortunately none of them took. So she came back begging me to do it again.

Again it was concert time 2013, and I went ahead and started with the injections and the whole procedure again. This time they harvested only 7 eggs of which only 5 were viable. They were inserted and we waited. She became pregnant with triplets and we were all ecstatic. She was over the moon. At 22 weeks, she was complaining of swelling in her legs. Her Gynae suggested she go to the chemist to have her blood pressure taken. It came back good and the Gynae said that all was okay and she must stay home.

At 24 weeks she started feeling abdominal pain and called her Gynae who said the same thing to her. That night she started bleeding and was rushed into hospital. The baby who was across her cervix had died and her body had started to go into labour to expel the dead foetus. This happens as the uterus grows, and the placenta gets pulled off as it was across the cervix. Once the placenta is not attached the baby no longer gest oxygen and dies. When it dies the body will go into labour to expel the dead foetus to prevent the body becoming toxic. Unfortunately because she was still pregnant with the other two it was a huge problem. She had to be admitted and they did an emergency caesarean to save the others. When they did this her bowels tore and her lungs collapsed and they had to work fast to save her life.

Because the babies were only 24 weeks old they were just too young to survive without severe mental or physical problems. 26 weeks most of the babies' organs and brain is developed enough to pull them through but 24 weeks is just not enough time. The one baby survived for a few hours and the other one for a day and then they were all gone. This was devastating for everyone. There were just too many things that went wrong for them to have survived.

She did survive, but underwent major surgery to her abdomen. This alone would take at least 6 months to repair if not longer. Her body was not ready to be exposed to another pregnancy and neither was mine. She however was desperate to try again and we waited exactly 6 months and then we started again with the procedure.

At this stage I started feeling that my body was tired, but very tired. I was feeling as if I needed to lie down a lot and that I was unable to exercise and I was just not my usually happy bubbly, busy self. So I suggested that we wait. I also said that 6 months was way too early for her to try again, especially after the major surgery she had gone through and the shock she had gone through both physically and emotionally. But she insisted and how can I say no after everything she had gone through. So we harvested again. This time there were 11 eggs.

As I was just too tired and not feeling happy or like I was having fun, I decided to go see an integrated health specialist. I told him that I was feeling very aggressive and very emotional. I would cry easily and was sitting in his office crying as I was telling him about the tiredness I was feeling. I didn't even have the energy to walk around the block and when my son begged me every day to walk around the block I would bribe him by saying, "Do you want a movie or walk around the block?" I knew he would choose the movie every time as we have a rule in our house that we only watch movies on Fridays and the rest of the week nothing. So to allow myself to lie on the couch and rest and not have to walk around the block I would offer him a movie. If he wanted to play outside a sword fighting game, I would offer to read to him a book on knights, again this meant I could lie on the bed and after two pages say, okay that's enough.

I was aggressive on the road, driving ridiculous speeds and if I got pulled over by the police I would question their authority and whether they had the right to stand on that corner and pull me over. Very unlike me, I didn't even have the energy to water my plants, so would just watch the pot plants suffering from lack of water and telling them to hold in there until the gardener got there in a few days' time.

Although I was always tired, I was not able to sleep. I would lie in bed for hours listening to my husband fall asleep and lightly snore his head off. I would check the time every now and then to see how late it was. Although I would be in bed by 9pm or earlier, I would still be awake at 12pm, waiting to fall asleep. Finally blissful sleep, but by 3 am I was awake again, waiting for the alarm to go off. With this I was experiencing all my pains. I had back pain, cramping on my front rib, cramping on my back, cramping calves and feet. I had restless legs, the dead arms, the sore hip and pain when I lie on my sides. I had rough patches of skin on my eyelids and face and knuckles, these were also sore and itchy at the same time, a form of eczema. I also had a blocked nose that clicked on the left when I spoke and when I menstruated I wanted to die because my bum bones felt like they were falling off. I would get sacral pain when I ovulated and I had severe pain in my sacrum when I bent forward or would do things on my hands and knees. Any position where my uterus was hanging would cause pain in my sacrum. But it was an organ pain and not a muscle pain.

I got the hormonal migraines any time I exerted myself in the form of exercise. I was tired of being tired to a point of being gatvol and there was nothing that I was doing that was helping. I had been eating healthily for 10 years and that didn't help. I was taking supplements and that didn't help. I was at my wits end. Even walking around the block would cause my body to become so stiff and sore the next day and this would last for days that it was just not worth the effort.

The Doctor drained my blood to do a plethora of tests and I was diagnosed with adrenal fatigue as well as a low Vit D. I started to research what it was about and how one treats it. The book called, *"Adrenal Fatigue: The 21st Century stress syndrome"* by James L Wilson, which a patient had come across and told me about brought a lot of insight and realization. In this book I was taught that adrenal fatigue is caused by a range of different things. These being: Trauma to the body or prolonged stress or a huge emotional shock. Chronic pain and depression can also result in adrenal fatigue. So basically anything that makes the body work hard over time or harder or on-going will result in adrenal fatigue. This made me realize that I was not the only one suffering from adrenal fatigue and most of my patients who were not responding to treatment, on closer examination of their blood, all came back with low cortisol levels, and low Vit. D levels indicating adrenal fatigue.

In my fourth year at university my dissertation was on Burnout and frankly I was now going through it. I had totally forgotten about this project and going through this made me stop and think about what we had said in the dissertation. The *"Adrenal Fatigue* "book also says that it is the disease of the 21st century and I can see it.

When I was reading the adrenal fatigue book it made a lot of sense. I had just asked my body to do 9 months and then 7 months and then 11 months' worth of work in a short period of time and then harvested its results. This is extreme for a body to handle. I realized at this point that my harvesting was the cause of the adrenal fatigue as I had not had fatigue and all these other funny symptoms like the hormonal migraines and increased pain prior to the harvesting. I was an epitome of health feeling happy energetic, pain free, apart from the odd kidney stone and enjoying life to the fullest, and then I harvested my eggs....

This was a huge drain on the system. Recently I decided to Google the side effects of harvesting your eggs. Much to my disgust they state there, No known side effects. But they fail to list the obvious side effects and the one on top of the list is: You reduce your child bearing years significantly and force your body into early menopause if you harvest your eggs. When women are born, we are born with a set number of eggs. When the eggs are finished you then go into menopause. When you reach menopause you then sit with all the other symptoms of hot flushes, mood swings, night sweats and irregular menstrual cycles that become shorter and then eventually stop. This means that you are no longer able to have any more of your own children.

By harvesting my eggs three times I reduced my child bearing years by 27 months, this is almost three years earlier. This is also just measuring the eggs that were harvested. However your body does not immediately go back to the normal rate of one egg per month after the hormones that were injected. I would have released more than one egg at a time, thus increasing the speed at which I was heading towards menopause and resulting in me going into Peri-menopause at age 40 instead of 50. This means that I my child bearing years have been significantly reduced.

So for 4 years I experienced Hormonal migraines, hot flushes, night sweats, mood swings and fatigue as well as severe pain when I ovulated especially on the left and pain during menstruation. To add to the irritation my hormonal cycle went to 21 days instead of 28 days. The fact that I have too much oestrogen in my body meant that I got gall stones and was diagnosed with osteopenia (my bones are thinning) and that's just from the hormonal side.

This has also affected my adrenal glands and I am still struggling to maintain the cortisol levels at the optimal level and they keep dropping down too low, and this causes the muscle pain, cramping, fatigue, poor sleep and aggression as well as a fat belly. So between the adrenal fatigue and the hormone imbalance I am a walking fire-breathing dragon that is confused and looking for the meaning of happiness, but couldn't be bothered to look too far because I am so tired I would rather just lie in a heap and feel sorry for myself and beat myself up with the invisible proverbial stick because I feel that I should be doing more.

Since that first time I have experienced the funny pupils on a not so regular basis but they come and go and it is a given that if I do any exercises like walking/running for 12km or dancing for 20min or swimming a race of 25 m, with a little more exertion than slow, that I will be man down within 30min of the activity for the rest of the day and night. Added to this I have the hot flushes, confused brain, forgetful brain and distracted brain. So I drive over big intersections when my light is red, and only realize what I am doing once half way over the road and honking horns are blaring at me. Horrors upon horrors, my angels are working hard in keeping me safe and have a bigger purpose in mind for me.

So what does all this mean and what do I need to do to correct it. Firstly, I should never have harvested my eggs, hind sight is a wonderful thing. But that is over and done and I can't turn back the clock. I can however inform every one that I know to not harvest their eggs, no matter what. It has also made me aware of adrenal fatigue and that it is present in many of my patients. It really is the illness of the 21st century and there is a way to treat it.

When I was doing my dissertation one of the recommendations that we made to prevent burnout/adrenal fatigue is to take 2 weeks off twice a year. Thus every 6 months you take off 2 weeks to recharge your battery and ensure you are always enjoying life to the fullest. This does not mean that you have to go away, you can quite happily stay home and just enjoy the time off to fiddle around the house and perhaps do some hobbies you haven't had the time to do, or frankly just lie and do nothing.

When I was diagnosed with the adrenal fatigue, I remember we went on holiday to the coast for 10 days. My husband was also diagnosed with adrenal fatigue so the two of us were both knackered. Each morning we would go to the beach and lie sleeping in the sun, while Vincent would attach himself to people who would be swimming in the sea. I always felt bad as the parents would scan the beach looking for the parent of this lost child, at which point I would raise my hand in a wave to say I am watching even though it is from far. Luckily Vincent is not one for going deep into the sea; he would just stand on the beach having the waves lap over his feet. Each day he would ask me if I could run on the beach or play with him or swim in the sea with him, so to placate him we would walk up the beach looking for shells for quite a while and then back to where we were lying, then I would have to tell him that I needed to charge my battery and that he must just play by himself.

He kept asking me if I was sleeping at night and when I said yes, he would ask me why my battery was not charged then. This made me think a bit, so I had to tell him that my charger was not charging properly and that was why I needed to charge it during the day too. He wanted to know how one could fix the broken charger and then I would tell him that I was taking special supplements that were designed to fix the broken charger. Again the "*Adrenal fatigue*" book mentioned that when you have adrenal fatigue that you need to specifically take adrenal extract to fix the problem. Thank goodness I was able to find a company that supplies a very good one and am having great results with my patients as well as myself. Your adrenal levels must be low though. So it is necessary to take a blood test to determine the levels.

In the beginning before my adrenal fatigue diagnosis, I would feel guilty about doing nothing. I would also feel guilty about not doing things with Vincent. Since I understand it a lot better, I no longer feel guilty about lying all day in bed if I feel like it. I also don't feel guilty about not walking around the block or lying watching TV. I know that my body needs to rest from time to time. I also know that I am generally an energetic busy body and when my levels are normal again I will get back to doing the normal busy things, but until then it's okay to lie around in a hammock sleeping and enjoying the birds twittering above my head. It is okay to spend a weekend lying in bed reading a good book and napping in between.

As I am writing this section it is overcast outside and raining after a long drought and I am feeling tired today. I have already spent an hour sleeping this morning when a patient cancelled and then I treated another patient and have a peaceful day the rest of the day. So I first thought that I wanted to lie and sleep again, but was not in the mood, so decided to do a little bit of hand sewing that now needs to be redone. I then decided that I wanted to do something but nothing too strenuous, and decided that writing this book was the perfect thing to do. I am not using up too much energy, but I am also productive. I want to get it done and I like to write and tell my side of the story, so it is a good thing to spend my time with.

I have many patients, who have adrenal fatigue. One of the ladies decided to take a 3 months sabbatical from work to recharge her batteries. She spent each day going to the gym for a light workout, she only woke up later in the morning when she felt rested and she took an afternoon nap each afternoon and made sure she went to bed early. She did not force herself to do anything strenuous. She did a little bit of light reading and decided to write on her own book. She was being kind to her body and did not feel guilty at all doing it as she knew she had to do it. After the three months, she decided that she would only work half day and focus on keeping her regime of exercising lightly and having a nap each afternoon. With this she continued to take her adrenal supplements and other supplements and focused on eating better. She still pops in from time to time to have a treatment, but her pain is under control and she has her old energy levels back and is feeling so much happier where she is in her life. She has also been able to resume her normal exercise regime of running and she has been able to take on more challenging tasks at work. She has learnt a lot and has informed me that she will never get into such a bad state again as she knows what caused it and thus avoids going into that cycle again.

One of my other patients who also suffered from severe fatigue also took a 3 month sabbatical, however she was so badly overworked from her previous job that she was not fully recovered even after the three months and is still struggling now with her health. She still has a long way to go, but with lack of work stressing her out now it's still draining her adrenal glands, but she has learnt a lot about what caused the problem in the first place and is thinking of implementing policies and procedures to protect the workers from having to go through the same experience. I believe that everything happens for a reason and these problems are brought across our path to make us stronger people and to put us in a position of knowledge that will enable us to help others to either avoid getting into a similar situation, or to help them overcome the same situation.

I think it is critical that people in general need to slow down. You need to make time to do what you are passionate about so that you can stay passionate about life and find joy in every moment of every day. Time is going by so quickly, that we need to make time to stop and smell the roses.

A few months ago I was treating another lady and her story is as follows. She would go to work every day earlier to avoid the traffic and then finish much later once again avoiding the traffic. She would also have an open door policy and because she is a loving caring person, she would have many of her personnel coming to her with their private problems asking for her advice. When she came to see me she was feeling over worked and underpaid. She had global pain in her body and was feeling burnt out. She did not want to take the pain medication as the side effects were worse than the actual beneficial effects of taking the pill and she was looking for an alternative means to get rid of her pain.

So we gradually went through the process of finding a balance of work hard, rest hard and play hard. In the first week she was able to leave work twice at the end of her work day and not stay later. This meant that she was able to walk around the block with her husband and get some exercise in. In the second week she was able to go home earlier (at home time) every day. Then we implemented that she has a closed door, so that she could be more productive during the day and only have her door open at certain times for people to come and talk to her. In the beginning the people ignored the closed door and still entered. I then suggested that she make a policy to help all people get more work done as she mentioned that productivity was down and so was morale. The policy would say something like: if the door is closed then you are working on a task and don't want to be interrupted, but that there would be certain times in the day that one could come and discuss personal matters or business matters.

The other problem she used to experience was that many people would come and talk personal matters towards the end of the day and then spend hours talking to her, making her leave late. I suggested that she tell them before they start talking that she only has 30min or an allotted time to talk to them and then if they need further time that they could schedule a proper time together later in the week when she would be able to talk to them properly.

I find if people know that you are interested in them but that you also have other commitments, then they don't mind if you only have 30minutes to talk to them, because they know you are prepared to listen to them at a later date as it has been scheduled in. Every body's time is valuable and we should treat it with respect. She has implemented everything that we have discussed and strategies we have come up with in our sessions. Because of this she is in a far better space and when she gets her pain, she knows exactly why. This is the most important part of the treatment. Life thrown her a curve ball and just as she was implementing all these good changes she was transferred to another building where she had to travel a lot further and this now takes back all the time we won. So we are back to square one with body pain and headaches, but we have a plan of action and hopefully by July her dream she wrote down when she did her goal setting, will materialize and she will be able to manage her own time and not be a puppet for someone else.

There was a book I read which had the following words *"If not me now, then who when*?" this made me really think about all the things we put off and procrastinate doing. If we have the attitude of if not me now then who when? We can achieve a lot more in our day. In this time we need to allocate time to exercise, time to be with the family and these times must be as important as going to work. Another saying I really enjoy saying to my patients is: "Start how you mean to end." When you start a new job, you are eager to prove yourself and eager to work long hours to be noticed. The problem comes in, is that when you offer your hand, they chew off your arm and when you look back in 3 years or 10 years' time, you will realize that you are all work and no play and are burnt out and hate your job and your life and there is no Joy in life, only work, work, work.

So when you start a new job, you work the hours you are being paid for and you continue with your social life and your gym and your family life as equal important times in your life. Never compromise, it's not worth it. If you inform your boss that you have an important meeting after work (gym) they will respect your boundaries and know that you mean what you say. Of course if there are deadlines and you need to stay after work for a few hours on the very odd occasion, that is okay, but it must never be the norm. That is NOT okay.

It is now quite a few years after my diagnosis and my energy is almost fully restored. I still need to take the supplements for a while longer, but my energy has enabled me to work for 3 weeks every day from 6h30 till 3pm in my garden, digging, planting, weeding, moving plants and statues and painting and mowing the grass. This was during my time off from work. As my gardener said to me, "Madam, you work like a Man!!" I am walking around the block with my son and sword fighting and dancing and things are really bright and I am having fun every day. My work is fun, my writing is fun, the walking is fun and great of all I am hitting more than 10 000 steps most days. I feel a thousand times better. I had the energy to redesign my back garden, and I have the energy to study further for the year. I have energy to read to my son and walk around the block without pain, and best of all, I have not wanted to watch TV at all. There are too many other things to do and I want to do them instead.

In loving Memory a poem I wrote after the death of the Triplets

The long wait for a miracle

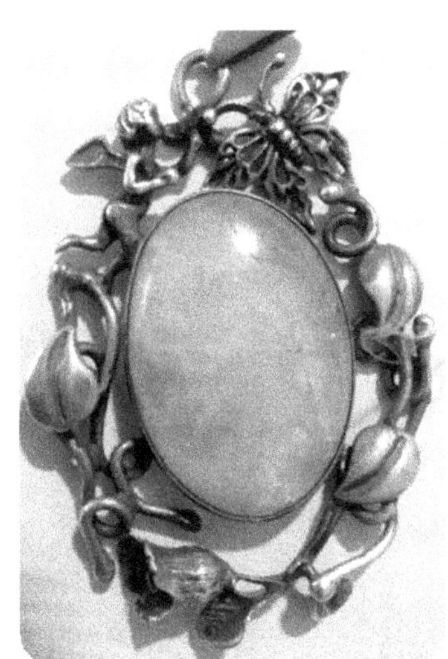

An Angel, butterfly and Rose,
All delicate and Pure,
Struggling for life, but unable to endure.

Let's remember these beings,
that brought so many feelings,
of happiness, hope and love.

But now we know they are safe in His
hands,
because of His plans
and will be fondly remembered.

Chapter 9
The 6 fundamental factors to being healthy

I mentioned earlier in the book about the nutrition course that I attended after being on the IMS course with Chan Gunn. I came across this course via a student that I had been supervising, who kept raving about this course. His brother kept telling him how good it was and how much he had learnt and this guy could not wait till he had funds and was finished with his physio degree to go on this course himself. I was not really paying much attention, as I was not really interested in learning about nutrition as I did not think it was relevant to my treatments. This was until I attended the IMS course.

Chan Gunn changed the way I thought about evaluating a patient. The fact that the student was constantly telling me about this Lifestyle course, I actually heard the statement Chan made. As I treat many patients with chronic pain, I come across a few who just don't respond to treatments. Now each time I go on a course these patients who do not respond are always on my mind and I am always looking for a reason as to why they are not responding. So when Chan said the following: *"If your patient does not respond to dry needling, then they have a metabolic problem,"* my ears pricked up.

He also said, that when you treat a patient, you have to evaluate the whole patient as looking at the area that is affected is not going to give you the solution. Often the muscle that supplies that area will be shortened and cause the problem, so if you release the entire muscle then you will see results. You also need to ensure that the entire body has full range in all areas, thus you need to treat the entire body.

He proceeded to show us how to evaluate each patient from head to toe and I have managed to take it further than just that by adding the information I learnt on the Nutrition and lifestyle coaching course.

When I got back to work on the Monday, I asked the student for the details on the diet course. And promptly went the following weekend on the course. Here they spoke about the 6 fundamental factors of being healthy. These explain why the people do not respond to dry needling or treatment and mostly it's because there is something other than a muscular problem that needs to be resolved. I mentioned in the previous chapter about adrenal fatigue, this is part of the metabolic problem. There is a deficiency in cortisol, or Vit D or Vit B or a range of other hormones and vitamins. Each one is very important for different functions in the body and depending on what the patient is complaining about, is what the Doctor will request blood tests for. Once the tests are back and the deficiency is noted, specific vitamins can be prescribed.

So the 6 fundamental factors are as follows:

1: Thoughts
2: Oxygen
3: Water intake
4: Food intake & supplementation
5: Exercise and
6: sleep

Out of these 6 factors, diet is the most important one and has the most radical change on your health and body, but if your mind is not with it and you are depressed, tired, unmotivated, don't know what to do, then it makes it a little hard to stick to doing the diet. You will be less likely to do what the therapist says. I have also noted that if you have a deficiency in your Vitamin D and a few other nutrients in your body, you will not be inclined to want to do exercise as you just don't feel well enough to do anything.

When I work with my patients, I always say to them that fixing the problem may require a number of different types of therapy. We need to work on their emotions doing tapping (EFT). We need to work on them physically and when they start feeling better, then we go into the next phase of doing the diet and drinking the correct amount and quality of water and lastly when you are feeling better then naturally you are going to want to be more active, and then we start adding specific exercises in. All these things will automatically improve your sleep and when everything has come together you will be feeling a lot better. When you are bad as most of my patients are, you need to start slowly. Sometimes it might even just be going to a therapist to reduce your pain.

So what do each of the 6 fundamental factors mean? Your thoughts are the most powerful aspect of your body. We are able to think ourselves sick and we are able to think ourselves well. There was a story I heard where a Doctor was doing a study on a placebo drug versus a drug used to treat cancer. One of the patients who had a huge tumour under his chin was allotted the placebo drug. When he took the drug, the Doctor told him that this magic pill was the answer to his prayers and that it would cure his cancer. This man had such faith in both the doctor and the pill that when he woke up the next morning his tumour had vanished and he was totally symptom free.

A few months later he heard via the newspapers that the drug he had been given was the placebo and the cancer returned the next day. When he arrived at the Doctors office, the Doctor told him that indeed he had been given the placebo drug but that the real drug did work and proceeded to give this man the same placebo drug, stating that it was the real thing this time. As in the previous time, his tumour disappeared by the next day and the man was cured. Telling you this story indicates how powerful the mind is and if it believes something this strongly it can overcome anything.

When I speak to my patients who suffer from depression, they tell me that it is a chemical imbalance and that there is no way they can heal and they will be on medication for the rest of their lives. I don't believe this always to be true. Yes I agree that they need the medication as they have not been given the tools to move forward and overcome the reason why they are depressed. If given the opportunity to do this and work through their emotional problems, then they may be able to reduce their medication as their coping strategies improve and they get a better understanding of why they are depressed and move on.

It was said in a news headline in the UK that more people have been given Prozac than the number of people who voted in Idols. This indicates that people have been given drugs when they don't necessarily need them. There are times when they are vital and one cannot do without them, so there is a place for them, but there are many different forms of help to improve your quality of life.

I do not state this lightly, but speak from my own experience. I too was depressed for about a year. I used to contemplate suicide in the form of driving off the road into the oncoming traffic or into a bridge. The only thing that stopped me was the fact that I had already had a car accident before and the outcome was extremely painful. So my thought process would be that if I did this and failed to kill myself that the pain and increased damage to my body could make my life a lot worse and in that case it was not even worth giving it a try. So I did the next best thing that I knew of and went to see a therapist. I only managed three sessions before I got so cross with her and myself. I was sitting telling her everything that I had been thinking of in my head for the past year and how bad my life was feeling, just because I had broken up with a longstanding boyfriend of 4 years. I felt like I was not going to find anyone else and that I was not good enough etc. etc. I would cry most of the time especially if I heard a sad song or thought of something sad and I would not laugh or make jokes. I felt alone and that no one noticed that I was feeling this bad.

After the third session she told me that I had two choices. The first one was that I needed to exercise. This was after my accident and when I exercised I would get severe headaches, so this was not really an option, and the second one was that I needed to take antidepressants. This made me so mad, as it felt like she did not hear what I had to say and neither option was acceptable to me at that time. At least fuming at this lady was better than being depressed and sad. When I reached home, my dad walked past me and told me to stop my nonsense. This took me by surprise as I told you it felt as if no one noticed me or realized that I was wallowing in depression. Even my brothers' dog would follow me around and when I sat down in my room, would sit and look at me with these woeful eyes and talk to me. When I walked he would take my fingers in his mouth and walk with me. For a long time I thought this was very peculiar, but later I realized he was trying to tell me something. Get over it and move on! He could smell the stench of depression.

Now I am not a dog person, more a cat person. I was a bit disturbed by this dog that kept following me around even though I am not the one that feeds him or gives him attention. I kept asking the dog what he wanted. We later discovered that this dog could smell diseases. When my sister brought her dog to the farm, Whiskey (this Labrador), would sniff his ear and drool incessantly.

So when my sister did a biopsy on the spot in the dogs' ear she found that it was cancerous. She removed it and the ear was fine.

The dog then kept sniffing the little dog's penis and drooling, so when we took the dog to the vet we were told the dog had a bladder infection. He got antibiotics and his bladder infection was cured and the dog no longer drooled. The dog sat by my mother when she was very ill and would sniff her and drool. She works as a physiotherapist in a children's ward, treating them for chest conditions and knew there was Influenza A going around and most of her patients were positive. So she knew that the dog was telling her that she was very ill and that she had also contracted this Virus. She was able to get medication to help her feel better as the dog had told her it was not just the common cold. If your dog is doing similar things, take note because they have much sharper intuition and noses than we do. Go have it checked out.

That same day after I had seen the therapist and was so mad I could spit snakes, I made a decision to get over my nonsense and get on with my life. The next day when I woke I was no longer depressed and I was able to move on and enjoy my life again. I saw this same reaction in one of my patients. She was a young woman who had attempted to commit suicide 35 times. Each time she would call her mother and tell her what she was about to do and then do it. Her mother would hurry to get to her side and then have to rush her off to hospital to have her stomach pumped or whatever else they needed to do depending on which means of suicide she chose that day. Her mother was in an absolute state of worry and depression and was so ill that she was physically unable to open her mouth big enough to eat. All she could fit in was a peppermint crisp, not the healthiest choice of food.

I by chance came across this patient when I was trying to take a photo of the sun with the rainbow around it and because it was so bright I had to move under a seated shaded area. I had to lean over this lady to take the photo. As I looked down at her I asked her if she was suffering from headaches as she looked like she was in pain. When she said she did, I then asked if she had been for physiotherapy which she said she had and that nothing was working. I asked if she had considered looking at her diet, which she said no. I offered her my card and said if she wanted to come that she was most welcome to call and I would see what I could do for her.

Both her and her mother became my patients and we worked on them for several months going through the different regimes I do. We did a lot of tapping with both of them and then the one session, she got so mad with me as I told her straight that she was being selfish as she was keeping her mother on a short leash and making her worried and ill. I told her if she wanted to commit suicide that she must get it over and done with so that her mother could stop worrying and if she doesn't really want to commit suicide that she must then stop her nonsense. Each time she tries to commit suicide she causes further damage to her body and increases her headaches and other pains in her body and I am not surprised that she is not getting better.

She swore at me and stormed out of my office and waited on the pavement for her mother to come fetch her. What I said must have triggered something in her like it had with me, as a few months later she called me to ask if she could come for a treatment, much to my surprise. When she came she had lost 10kg and her headaches were much less intense. She was in the neighbourhood to go for a job interview and was super excited as she had not been able to keep a job because of her illness and headaches. She reported that she no longer had the urge to commit suicide and was feeling a lot better inside. I recently heard from her again and she informed me that she was now married and has just had a little girl and is doing really well.

You are going to get a chemical imbalance when you are depressed and the more negative thoughts you have the more chemicals your body will release to keep this going. This is why it is so important to make a conscious decision to have a good day every day. It is hard to get the ball on the move and you will need someone to help nudge you in the right direction or in my case and this case above, make you so mad that you make a decision to get better and do what you have been told to do. I have found the EFT for this is invaluable and I will discuss this in a lot more detail. The EFT really makes your mind open to other possibilities that you have not even considered.

I was working with one of my patients using the EFT technique for her depression. We were talking about how changing your perspective on things using the EFT can make you feel happy and lighter and resolve your depression. She then asked me a most profound question and maybe you have this same feeling. She asked me what it felt like to be happy as she could only tell me how it felt to be depressed as this is the only feeling she knows since she was a little girl, and she wanted to know, how she will know, in a normal day, if she was happy and okay. This is a vital question and one that I pondered for 6 months myself, when I came up with the following understanding.

At the beginning of 2016 I was wondering why it felt like I had no joy in my life. I came to the conclusion that I enjoyed playing sport, dancing, being active and feeling my lungs burn from the exertion of exercise and doing these things with people. So I broke it down to: "I like being active and doing things with people." My next question then was: What am I doing currently that fits this description? My answer to that was: I am doing the belly dancing and that I enjoyed working with my patients. So my next question was: "If I am doing something that should be fun, then why is it not fun?" I then changed the way I thought about the whole thing. My way of thinking then turned to: "when dancing is fun again, I will know that I am better and that my body has healed."

So then my patient asked. "How will you know you are having fun and that you are better, what will you feel like?" And to this I said: "When you bop to the music on the radio and hum to the song or sing with, when you feel calm enough to sit and watch the fish swim in a pond and to walk in the garden and enjoy the birds singing. When you feel the urge to do more things on a daily basis like go to the shops and admire some paintings or pop into the shops you used to like going to. Or you feel like Googling a song you heard because it was so nice. Or you feel like walking around the block or doing some exercise classes at home using You Tube. Then you know you are happy and having fun. It's not the special events of going to a show, but the daily things that you do, and how you feel when doing them.

Is it a drag to do activities and all you want to do is lie down and not cook or clean and do nothing, while beating yourself up mentally for being a lazy slob? Or are you doing the normal day to day things while humming your favourite song and dancing?"

Which one do you want it to be?

When I told her this, she was feeling much happier, because she had a picture in her mind as to where she needed to move towards and knew what her picture would look like when she had arrived. Again, once you know what the finish line looks like, you are able to knuckle down and work on the mundane day to day challenges like doing the tapping, eating correctly, taking your supplements, going to bed early and doing some form of exercise. Remember not all at once but as you feel better you will want to do more and it's a gradual process and an amazing journey of learning who you are and what you want and like and what makes you happy. It's really worth the effort.

I have touched on some patient stories where they needed some EFT to help them move forward in their lives and eradicate the pain which was caused by the emotional upheaval. Now I would like to show you how to do it yourself. Over the next few chapters, we will go into details through each of the fundamental factors.

Chapter 10

Changing the way you think through EFT

Many of us have experienced a range of different experiences throughout our lives. Most of these experiences are linked with a range of different emotions from good to bad. When I speak to my patients, some of them have a despair that has been created by their long standing problems. These patients have been from Doctor to Doctor looking for answers to their pain and have been to so many places with no resolution to their problem that they get depressed thinking that their life will be like this for ever.

Some patients start with despair or even depression due to emotional circumstances from when they were young or events that were very traumatic for them. They feel a deep hate towards themselves and towards life and struggle to cope with day to day living. This uncertainty and depression then creates physical problems such as headaches and back or hip pain. These patients will not have had a physical injury, but will also go from Doctor to Doctor looking for a solution, but all the scans will come back clear, the blood results may be normal and thus they continue in a cycle of depression not knowing how to break it down and swim to the surface.

These experiences shape the person you are today, but many of these feelings such as depression, no longer serve a purpose, but actually hold you back from becoming the best you, you can be. Many of these people have been for counselling and the problems they have been thinking of have been going round in their head over and over. They have thought of all the different scenarios and know that there is no real solution to the problem, it is what it is, which is why they feel so bad. When one has these thoughts stuck on repeat, it can influence your concentration and short term memory as the brain is constantly trying to think of a solution to the problem.

At the beginning of the book I asked that you complete your time line. This time line indicates when physical problems started such as depression, fatigue, pain, headaches etc. If you did not have a physical injury during that time period when the problem started, then you need to see if you were going through a difficult or stressful situation. It can be anything from getting married, to having a baby, to the negative of going through a divorce or a death of someone dear and close to you. Even living in a difficult home environment and moving often or living with an alcoholic parent can cause trauma in your life. Anything can set the body into a spiral of disease or pain.

To repair this disease and pain we need to change the way you think of the whole situation. I mentioned that one of the most important aspects of healing is having the right frame of mind. Once you have this, you will be able to take on anything and change your life. Einstein said you can only improve yourself if you change the frame of mind in which the problem was created. Often we still feel the same and think the same as we did when we were injured or went through the difficult situation. By changing the way you think about this problem you can change the outcome.

When I was in the UK there were a number of patients whom I treated with huge emotional issues. The first was a lady in her forties. She came to me with a pain in her hip and after every treatment was pain free, but when she returned the next session, her pain was exactly the same as it was when I first saw her. During the treatment sessions, she went away for a week on holiday and reported that when she drove towards the holiday destination, her hip pain went away but when she drove back home, the hip pain returned. This information lead me to believe that it was stress related and we were able to target a different approach to treatment. Once she realized that her pain was due to stress and that she was unhappy, we could change the way she thought about her situation and with this we were able to resolve her hip pain.

The second was a patient who was complaining of such severe back pain that his posture was pulled to the one side. We call it a list. The MRI scan was clear and there was no evidence of injury, and there had been no injury. He too responded well to treatment and got off the bed feeling great but when he returned he was exactly the same. After the third session I started quizzing him as to what was bothering him and to tell me exactly what he was doing when the pain first came on. He reported that his back went into spasm when he was getting out of the car at his fathers' funeral and that he did not want to be there. The last time he had seen the family was when they had buried their grandfather and they had left on bad terms and had not spoken to each other since then.

He also reported that he was stressed at work and at home, as they had just moved house and his wife was pregnant with their first child. He had been promoted to a manager of 40 people and his brothers' child was diagnosed with a terminal illness. So many things were going on in his life. When I told him that it was stress related he didn't want to believe me. So he went home and did what everyone does: Google: he found a booked called *"Healing back pain, the mind body connection"* by John E Sarno. In this book the author tells people how stress can cause all kinds of pain and that one needs to continue with your normal daily work as activity does not actually change the intensity of the pain. You cannot let the pain get the better of you and start worrying yourself in to an even sicker state.

So he gradually started being more active and the more active he became the less pain he experienced. I taught him relaxation techniques and if I had only known about the EFT back then, I am sure we would have had results much quicker. As mentioned several times, once you know what the problem is and what is causing the pain, then you can tackle the problem head on and resolve it.

Another lady I treated was a refugee from Iraq who had been held in captivity by Sadam Husein himself. She was forced to sit in a crouched position for 2 weeks in a small box. She was only given just enough water to survive and had to sit in her excrement. When I evaluated her she was complaining of extreme pain in all her joints, but there were no injuries on the X-ray reports or anything wrong in her blood works, but the extreme circumstances led me to believe that this was due to huge amounts of fear and stress as well as the poor circulation from sitting crouched. So I taught her relaxation and did guided meditation with her. Again if I had known about the EFT technique I think she would have benefitted hugely.

I have treated patients' who have been abused by family members or people in trusting positions such as headmasters, priests, their own father or brothers and uncles. All of them were depressed and overweight and all of them suffered from headaches and global body pains. These pains will not go away unless the entire person is treated holistically. One needs to work on the emotional issues at play as well as the physical problems that have been created due to the emotional aspects. Most of these patients have been to see psychologists and psychiatrists and are on a range of medication that makes them feel like walking zombies. Their emotions are dumbed down but they still don't feel better. They are used to talking about their problems and rattle them off like a story, but with EFT we need to approach it differently. If they are going to rattle off the story we are not going to get the deeper understanding and it's not going to work because one goes off on a tangent and circumvent the lesson or meaning one may have learnt from the situation. You also don't get to change the way you think about the situation.

EFT has the most amazing results with patients. One uses specific points on the body that give you access into the subconscious. The nice thing about the brain and the not so nice thing about the brain is that it can't tell the difference between reality and fantasy. So when you relive the memories, the same chemicals are released which increases the heart rate and makes you feel helpless or powerless or scared. It's the same when you watch a horror movie or have a dream.

If however we change the memory, the brain then releases a different hormone and the body believes that this is actually what happened. The body relaxes and the person actually feels more relaxed and calmer about the experience. Often they say it feels like a weight has been lifted off their shoulders or that it feels like they were watching a movie.

What I say to my patients, is that if you are depressed, or angry or anxious or whichever emotion we are working on, that it will be a forest of that emotion. Each tree in the forest is symbolic of an event that occurred which strengthens this emotion. For example, if the person is depressed and thinks they are worthless, so have a low self-esteem, due to feeling unloved and uncared for as a child, or even abused as a child, every time they were abused, or hurt, a tree would have been planted to make your feeling stronger. So if your life has been rather tough, your forest will be quite thick. Alternatively, you can have such a traumatic single event, that this single event can over shadow any other event overriding the previous belief totally. Most of our beliefs are created within the first 7 years of our life, so often traumatic events in this time of your life will have huge repercussions in your life.

When we work with EFT, we take each memory of one of these events and pause it in the mind. We analyse the feeling involved and we give it a rating out of 10 where 0 is no problem or anger or depression and 10 is so bad you want to commit suicide or you want to do nothing in life. Some of my patients even say that the event is 20/10 as it just feels worse than anything they have experienced before.

One will then just tap on the side of the hand and repeat the words *"even though I am depressed/sad/anxious/lonely...., I am okay and I would like to accept myself anyway."* You repeat this three times. You can elaborate and add to the sentence the feelings that come up inside, such as. "even though I was hurt and unable to defend myself and hate being depressed and that there are so many times I have felt this way that I do not know how else to feel, I am okay and would like to accept myself anyway."

Some people when they say "I am okay and would like to accept myself" feel uncomfortable saying this because they do not believe this to be true. They are not okay. They are suffering from severe headaches and depression and are not their happy normal selves. So, no, they are not okay. And frankly with all the things they have been through, they aren't able to accept themselves. So one would then change the words to "even though I am feeling depressed and I am not okay, I would like to move forward to being okay and being able to accept myself anyway." This way the brain does not rebel against what you have been telling it for years. How can it be okay when you have been telling it for years you are NOT okay?

By changing the wording slightly the brain accepts it and believes it to be true and before you know it, you are saying things like "actually I am okay and I am alive and not dead so I must be okay, I am not great, but I am okay”. The amazing thing about these words is that we are confirming and acknowledging what we believe and what we have been through.

Most of the time there is nothing one can do about the past or the future, but yet we worry about it all the time. Our mind gets stuck on a spin cycle that never ends. This makes us unable to concentrate properly. We speak about the same things over and over and still feel just as bad about them and don’t know how to move forward. Or we don’t talk about them and let the thoughts fester inside our bodies and allow these stressful thoughts to cause headaches and body pains.

The body is very sneaky. Even when we do the tapping and you have an epiphany that stress is causing your headaches, the body will try and derail you and sabotage your thinking by causing back pain instead of headaches and one needs to keep on your toes and realize that the body is trying to get attention again. If you resolve the issue as to why you are feeling that specific feeling, then the body does not need to find another spot to cause pain, because you have resolved the underlying issue.

If you do not find the correct words or the correct feeling then the area will not release. I have a patient who apart from having pain everywhere has pain specifically in her jaw from clenching her teeth. We have tapped before for the jaw and it did not release. She would keep saying that “everyone says the jaw is stress related, but I don’t think so.” So when I asked her what she thought it was caused by, she thought about it for a few minutes before answering: “From having to keep my mouth shut and not say what I desperately want to say because I know I will get shouted at for saying it.”

She has a very strong moral compass and does not like it when some people are favoured above others. She feels she is required to stand up for these people and inform the person who is doing the wrong behavior that this is not acceptable even if she has nothing to do with the situation. This unfortunately has back fired a number of times in her face and then she feels even worse and gets cross, because how can things be so wrong. Sometimes, it's not the fact that we stand up for the people, but what comes out of our mouths that upsets them. If you have this urge to speak out, then you need to learn to become very diplomatic. I read a book that said you must sandwich the bad between the good.

If for instance there is a problem at work and the staff are unhappy. You would then in a meeting point out what works well. Then you would point out what was not working, which is why the staff is unhappy and then you could make a suggestion that could help resolve the issue. Perhaps mentioning what the staff has already said works well with them would be adequate.

By getting to the nitty gritty of why her jaw was always clenched, and recognizing it and acknowledging that it is a right behaviour but that we need to work on the presentation thereof, altered her thought processes and released the jaw instantly. It's all about clarity and once again the clenching of the jaw was not helping her situation, in fact it is causing more pain. Now in future situations where she feels the need to speak up for others, she may think twice about how she is going to present it and also she probably won't get as angry about the situation as she did in the past as this did not serve her properly. Remember though that this jaw is a forest of anger and it may release at that moment in time, but it can also return if there are other underlying issues that have still to be resolved.

I told her the story of when I was working in the UK as the head of a department. Every Friday my superintendent would come to the hospital for the morning and see what was going on. In the UK the people there are very sarcastic it's their culture. In South Africa, sarcasm is used to be nasty and rude. So each Friday she would come to the department and drop sarcastic remarks all morning. I assumed she didn't like me and thought I was not doing a good job and this resulted in me going home every Friday night and crying because I'm not loved. It took four years for me to pull up my socks and approach her. I was dreading it, because if I did things like that in the past I would forget what I wanted to say. I would not be able to find the right words and I would not be able to express myself properly and then I would cry. I hated this about myself, so was adamant that this was not going to happen. So I prepared for the meeting and wrote down everything that she said that offended me and how it made me feel.

The next Friday I went with my note book and I asked her if she was available to chat somewhere private. I whipped out the pad and asked her directly if she had a problem with me and if she didn't like me. She looked at me astounded and asked me why I thought such things. I read off the little sarcastic remarks she always said. She was taken aback and told me that she was unaware that this made me feel like that and that she would never say those things again. She considered me to be a valuable staff member and I was doing a great job and that she wanted me to stay as long as I wanted to be there. Now I was shocked by her reply as it really was not as bad as I had thought it would be. This also made me realize that many people feel the same way and have the same situations at work. I vowed from then on to make sure I speak my mind with clarity and to make sure I think about what it is that I want to say before the time, so that I do not forget and cry. I have become very sharp in my negotiations with people and am not scared any more.

Tackle your fear head on and make your own list. Many people I have told this story to have followed suite and have had just as amazing results as I did. It makes such a huge difference. You are not an underdog that can allow other people to walk all over you. You don't have to be nasty about it, but you are allowed to speak your mind and feel okay about it. Again the phrasing is very important. You will always say it as "I feel very sad/hurt/angry/shocked etc. when you (do or say the negative thing)........."

Make it all about you and not about them, then they won't get their hackles up.

To make things easier I have taken the EFT cheat sheet[pg144] from my mentor, who taught me the EFT technique, with her blessings. Here you can clearly see the areas you tap on the body and the wording that needs to be said.

Now you have been tapping on the emotion of depression 8/10 and during the tapping find that it is reducing to 4/10 and then 2/10 until you are able to get it to a 0/10. This often occurs within the same treatment sessions. When we take a specific memory from childhood, we will then change it to make it feel better. If it is not shifting then you may be working with the wrong memory or wrong emotion, but you will still feel better and you will still get results as the body will accept any EFT as good and emotions will still shift.

Perhaps you would like an adult you trust to enter the picture and speak soothing words to you (in your mind), or if there is no such adult, then perhaps a faithful Angel could help with the task at hand. I like to use the picture of Angels, they are so calming and can fold their wings around you or fly you up into the clouds leaving the body behind to go through the experience, but the soul is safe and having a totally different experience. This is called matrix re-imprinting. The interesting thing about this is that if you can find the main memory that is holding all the depression in place, you can remove it.

Basic EFT Technique

Step 1: Choose a problem to work with

Step 2: Rate your anxiety or discomfort (where 0=no distress and 10=highest level of discomfort) when you think about it right now. (How anxious are you? How uncomfortable do you feel?) Also, close your eyes, check in your body and feel where you feel it in your body.

Step 3: Tap the karate-chop point (on the fleshy side of the hand) while you say the problem and then finish by saying that you're still ok: *Even though I have this [problem], I deeply and completely love and accept myself.* Repeat 3 times.

Step 4: Tap on each of the following stress-relief points while repeating a short reminder of the problem (for instance "this fear in my stomach")

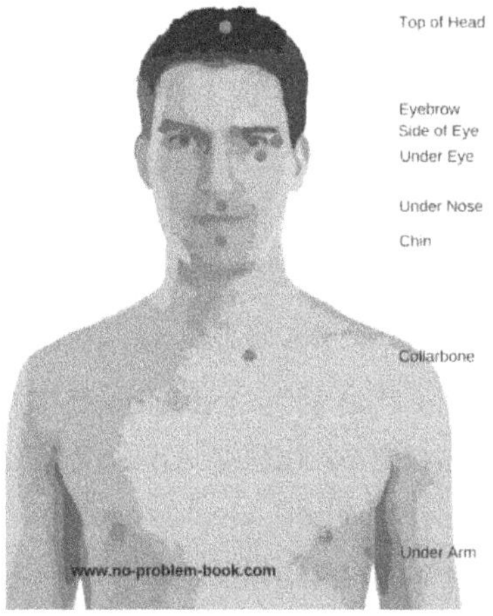

Step 5: Rate your anxiety or discomfort again. If any discomfort remains, repeat the steps above until you're down to a 0. You can adapt the Set-Up Statement (Step 3) to "Even though I still have some fear of...."

Step 6: If you're not making headway, there is a variety of trouble shooting options. Please contact me for assistance.

Liesel Teversham www.no-problem-book.com liesel@no-problem-book.com

***Taken from "No problem" by Liesel Teversham published by KIMA books**

There was a story that was told at the course where we were learning to do the matrix re-imprinting. The lecturer was telling us of one of his patients who was diagnosed bipolar and would often have depression cycles that would last weeks, with few happy cycles. During the session, she went into her depression as it was activated by a core memory. As they discussed the core memory and changed it to a memory that was more acceptable, the depression lifted and she totally felt free. She later reported that her depression had not returned and that she was able to stop all medication.

I have seen this happen in my practice. I had a lady who was booked off work due to anxiety and not being able to cope in normal day to day living. She had been like this for 2 years prior to seeing me. On her first evaluation I asked her if I could do needling with her for her neck pain and she totally fell apart, crying about the thought of me doing needles with her. It turned out that the previous session she had with needles with another therapist had caused her to have an autonomic reaction where she got the shakes after treatment at home. It was so bad that she thought she was dying and she had this intense fear of going through that again. I did two tapping sessions with her and at the third session she reported that she was no longer anxious and that she wanted to try the needles again. Not long after that she was totally pain free, no longer had panic attacks and was able to return to work. It was amazing.

When one does the tapping with a therapist, you get the most amazing AHA moments. It brings such clarity to you that you are able to move forward because it brings acceptance. The whole reason why one is depressed or anxious is because you feel unsafe and unloved and don't know what to do to change this. When you get clarity as to why things have happened in your life, you are able to close the door on the chapter. I do find the analytical people difficult to treat this way as they are not very open to weird airy fairy techniques and think it is a waste of time and don't like opening up to the experience.

I shifted a lot of baggage in the 6 months I did the EFT, every week logging into Skype and spending an hour to 2 hours tapping on my problems and emotions. From Anger, to sadness, to tiredness, to hate and all these emotions came bubbling up. My aggression that

I had been struggling with lifted totally. I felt light and free and felt that I was starting to have joy in my life again. This is when I did the soul searching of what is Joy in my life. When I found the joy in my belly dancing class, I celebrated by making belly dancing skirts and new bras and belts all done up with feathers and bling.

I took it a step further as I was feeling extremely creative and designed my own head piece of feathers. I asked the dance instructor if we could do Rio the movie and look like birds on stage. I designed feather arm pieces or tails and wings to complete the costume. We don't have the music yet or the dance moves yet, but I don't really mind, as it was fun doing it and just being creative and a little mad. I not only made one head piece, but enjoyed it so much I made 3, one for every skirt I happened to have. I took these head pieces and displayed them in my home over the Christmas period. It was so pretty and colourful and there were feathers everywhere. My cats also agreed with me that it was beautiful. My husband jokingly asked if he should get me a mannequin to display the pieces on, and I rather thought that it was a very good idea.

If he can admire his minis reflection in the shop window while he drives past in the street, then I can admire my work on a mannequin.

At the end of the year I went for 4 one on one sessions via Skype. This I did to clear things that had happened in the year and close the year off well. I cannot tell you how refreshed and energized I have felt over December and January. I even have enough patience and energy to sit and do homework with my son of Grade 4.

I have not been able to tolerate doing any homework with him since Gr1 as it was just too frustrating. He has been very good and has done it all by himself. But he can do with a little guidance with his maths and now I have the patience to help him. So we have gone and bought some extra Maths books for both grade 3 and grade 4 and have managed to do our first two pages together and I did not lose my cool even once and it took us some time as he was rather confused as to what he needed to do. This little bit of attention has helped him understand a few things quite quickly; it just needed to be explained to him in a different manner.

When I was at school I was really good at helping teach the others in the class how to do Maths or biology as I do enjoy teaching. It was rather strange that I could not tolerate this at all, but I know it was all to do with the adrenal fatigue and I can move on and do a better job this year.

I felt very silly in the beginning when I was doing the tapping. You are going to feel silly too, but the results are too good to ignore this technique.

In the goal setting chapter I spoke in depth about what you want and how to think about getting it. For many years I have been writing down my dreams and goals at the end of the year in preparation for the next year. This has been really amazing as when I take it out at the end of the following year, I cannot believe how much I have achieved. This is very important in getting your mind thinking in a more positive direction and to eradicate the negative thoughts. When you have improved your thoughts and changed the way you feel about the past, you will be able to set new habits that will improve your future way of thinking.

There was a book I read that states you must spend 10min per day thinking about your day, 1 hour a week, one day a month and one week a year. So during the time that I am on holiday at the end of each year I spend this time thinking about what I want to do, be or have in the coming year. Then each morning when I wake up I focus on what I want to achieve for the day and what I would like to have happen. Then at night I spend a few minutes while lying in bed drifting off to sleep being grateful for everything that happened in the day and everything that I have achieved and received.

I read that, the more you are grateful for then the more you will be given to be grateful for. This is very powerful and so true and I believe it to my core. The other thing one must do is write down 100 things you wish to be, do or become. The goal chart at the beginning of the book helps you get your mind on the right track to do this.

The one year I wrote down the following goals. I wanted a house between Johannesburg and Pretoria so that commuting would be easy in both directions. The house must be an old house with a big garden and it must be in a safe area. It must have big rooms and a long passage, like the old houses in South Africa all have. It must be able to be changed so that I can easily work from home. It must have a driveway to the side of the house that goes to the back of the house with a garage big enough to work in and park the cars in. It must have a swimming pool and it must have a big blank canvas for a garden.

Secondly I wrote down that I wanted an Audi 1.9 TDI, with 60 000km on the clock and that I must be able to pay cash for it. It must be either silver or gold. Thirdly I wrote down that I wanted to be pregnant with my first child. At the end of the year when I took out the folded piece of paper I had everything that was on that list.

The house we bought is found in Centurion, it was built in 1973 so has the old strong structure, long passage, big garden with swimming pool and the previous people did not garden, so blank canvas. The garage can house two cars and in our case three minis and it has a work area where my husband can tinker on the cars and do what he loves to do. It also has maids' quarters with a bathroom. Soon after we moved in we renovated the house, as it still had the old carpets from 1973 and smelled a bit stale when it rained.

The house did not feel like home, the previous owners had 8 foster children who used to smoke in the rooms as there was evidence of cigarette butts on the windowsills and in the cupboards in all the rooms. The sewage drains were totally blocked. The people also used to bury their rubbish in the back garden, when there is rubbish removal.

It was not long before we had a new home, redone inside with new flooring and new paint and a few alterations to enable me to work from home. We made the long passage shorter by enlarging the one bedroom to become the main bedroom and the main bedroom became my work room by adding an external door to access the room from outside. We added a second gate and a parking area for my patients to park safely inside. The garden became an area that was used to its fullest potential as before there were certain dead areas that never got used. The few surviving indigenous plants got moved to the correct place and many other indigenous plants got planted to create a haven for the little birds and other creatures.

As for the car, I got an Audi 1.9 TDI with 58 000 on the clock and I paid cash for it. It was Champagne colour, so a combination of both silver and gold, and I was pregnant with my first child.

As you get in tune with writing down your goals and expecting them to happen, they start to happen even quicker. After we had redone the house I went on a garden design course, as I wanted a stunning garden that attracted lots of bird life and wild animals. I planned it out on paper and started the long process of digging and planting. The one day I was thinking that I needed to get some rocks to elevate a flower bed. I phoned my mom who lives on a farm and asked if I could borrow the bakkie and come and fetch rocks for my garden. However the bakkie was out of commission for the week so I would have to wait. The very next morning I heard this banging noise from over the road. It was my neighbour who was throwing away his rocks that had been lying around in his garden for the past 25 years when they had dug their swimming pool. So I got my rocks with no effort and delivered to my doorstep. I used the rocks throughout my garden to lift more than one flower bed. When I had done that I was in need of soil. I was thinking about where I would need to order soil from, when one of my patients asked if she could pay me in horse manure instead of cash. I immediately agreed and my soil arrived the same week.

Now all I needed was agapanthus to plant in the flower bed. So once again I contacted my mom to ask her if I could come dig some out. But before I could get out to the farm, my neighbour two doors down, asked if she could borrow my gardener to come and dig out her agapanthus and replant them as there were too many and I was welcome to have the left overs.

This is really true. The more you write down what you want, the more you will get what you ask for. If you do not ask or do not know what you want, then how must your body or your subconscious know what you want? Once you have written things down and you become more grateful for what you have, things just start falling into place.

These past few years I was not able or not in the mood to go through my yearly goal setting due to my adrenal fatigue. I just did not have the energy, I felt quite lost and felt that I was just going through the motions of life and waking every day to work and lie and sleep and repeat the cycle over and over. I felt that the joy had been sucked out of my life and I did not know what fun was anymore. I felt that I had lost touch with my Spiritual IQ and that nothing was going my way, even though it was not that bad really. Yes my health was a bit suspect, with the low energy, but my work was good. I felt stressed and felt like I was having no fun and I felt confused in my brain. There was no goal and nothing driving me forward apart from what I had to do on a daily basis. I was bored but I was tired, so it was okay, but my brain was thinking of all these ideas, but I had no energy to implement any of them and I was not myself.

I was at a course where the speaker was talking about Mental IQ, Physical IQ, Emotional IQ and Spiritual IQ. This is where all my confusion in my brain made sense to me and I had the light bulb effect go on. She stated that you are born with a specific IQ and by learning to do a certain task you are working on your physical IQ. So yes you can improve your physical IQ by practicing more and becoming good at what you do. If you however work on your emotional IQ by reading self-empowering books and learning how to control your emotions and work on how you react in certain situations, then you will increase your effectiveness 3 times more than just learning how to do the work, which is the physical IQ and having the mental IQ.

If however, you become grateful for what you have and aware of what you want and tune into your quiet space and prayer, then your possibilities become infinite. So you tune in to your spiritual IQ and then there is no holding you back as things just fall into place. You get your dream house, your dream car, the rocks, soil and plants. This is what happens when you tune into your Spiritual IQ. So my ah ha moment was realizing that since I had not been spending quiet times going through my goals for the year and I had not been spending 10 min a day thinking about what I wanted to happen for the day, I was not in tune with my spiritual IQ and that is why life was feeling really hard and tough at that moment in time.

I had not taken time to rest and be quiet in a meditative way, or in prayer. I was not getting the results that I usually get and this was frustrating and not me or my life. This was all because I was not in tune with the spiritual aspect of life and if I just took the time to become quiet on a regular basis, then things would fall into place and voila things would start happening. You don't need to work harder to get better results, you need to find a balance between rest hard, work hard and play hard.

I have many of my patients and even my son tells me that they feel like they don't belong. Vincent (my son) often says, "Mommy it doesn't feel like I belong in Grade 3 or in the school where I go". So my question is: If you don't belong there, then where do you belong? One of my patients told me the same thing. So when I asked her, if you don't belong there, then where do you belong? She thought a bit and then told me, I guess I belong where I am. Every decision you make or your parents make leads you to be where you are at this moment in time doing what you are doing. It is an active or sometimes a passive decision and if you do not like where you are because you are not happy, then change it. Choose where you want to be and find your passion and make yourself feel like you belong. You need to feel that you are appreciated.

I worked at a hospital in the children's ward where the nursing staff loved having me there as they used to say that I did a good job and the children always got better. However I did not feel appreciated by the Doctor. We then got a newly qualified Dr who informed me in no uncertain terms that I was not allowed to communicate with the patients and that it was her job to give advice to the patients. Now as a physiotherapist we are first line practitioners and we are educated enough to be able to give sound advice on what the patient needs to be able to do to get better.

I thought about the situation and within a short period I had made a decision to no longer work in an environment where I was not appreciated. I informed the sisters that I would find a physio to take my place, but that I was no longer available to work in the hospital. I professionally informed the Doctors that I was moving forward with my practice in another direction and that I would no longer be available to help them with their patients. It was the best decision I have ever made.

During this period of time my mother was looking into retirement or scaling down. She is also a physiotherapist and works in a children's wards treating only kids with pneumonia and other chest conditions. From time to time I have been there to help her out, so I know the sisters that work there. She has mentioned several times to me that when she retires, that I can gladly take over her practice. So when I was making all my other decisions in life and wondering what fun was and what the point in life was, I came across a book which told me to do the following:

Like to	Love to
Hate to	Have to

In this quadrant you analyse your life according to the quadrant. This made a huge difference in my life. As I mentioned, my mother wanted me to take over the work at her hospital. Now this would be a very lucrative business and I am guaranteed payment. So I thought about what I loved and liked about my work. I came to the conclusion that I liked what I currently was doing and when I looked at what I didn't like and what I had to do, I thought about working at the hospital. To elaborate: My work at home is with people who suffer from chronic pain, basically going through what I have already gone through and thus I know what I am doing and what I am teaching as I have been there, and got the T-shirt. So I get to know my patients well and know what they are feeling, thinking and doing and together we move forward on the journey of health. This is such a great feeling when you can see the progress and see them change into people who feel amazing and think differently to how they used to think.

My work in the kids ward is brain dead work, because there is no challenge. They are all in for chest conditions of pneumonia or bronchitis or a sinusitis, so there is no real thinking needed. But it is also stressful. The reason why I find it stressful is that I will have a full day at home and be quite happy treating my patients there and the hospital will phone and say. “By the way, there is a child here for you to come and see.” The first thing that irks me is the words: “By the way.” I get the impression they think I am waiting around doing nothing, hoping they will call me to come and work. The second thing that gets me boiling is that I have to find time to squeeze the treatment into a full day. I fetch my son when school finishes, but I drive past the hospital. So either I must call the school to tell him I am going to be late, and then stop and treat the child, or I must fetch him and he comes with to the hospital and waits while I treat the child. Either way, I feel guilty because I know he hates the hospital and secondly I know he hates to wait for me at school.

Neither option will kill him or do him any harm, but my guilt chews me up and I feel super rushed and stressed. Then I will arrive at the hospital and there won’t be one child but sometimes up to five. This is a good two hour’s work excluding travel time. Now my conscience would prick me too much if I did half a job, so I grin and make jokes and no one is any the wiser that I am boiling with fury underneath. But I am worrying about my son, as I will no longer be 20 minutes late, but two hours late and then we are going to get stuck in the traffic.

This is not good for my health. Then to top it all off, you get the parents who are worried about their children, but they accuse you of doing things that are not true, or create havoc in the ward or are so rude to you, you wonder why you even bother to treat their child. They get the impression that just because they are paying for your service, that they can talk rudely to you or even swear at you, when you have no idea what it is you have done wrong, because you have just arrived to treat their child.

I do not need that in my life, and then they turn around when the medical aid refuses to pay and say they were never at treatment. This just baffles me that people can be so crude and nasty. I had been pondering taking over my mother's hospital practice, where I would have to treat kids every day. I would be exposed to those nasty germs, and it is a guarantee that I will get sick on a regular basis working with them. I would not be able to do my work at home which I love. I would have to treat the hospital kids every day and if there is no one to work on the weekend or on a public holiday, then I would have to work. I have watched my mom over the many years working at the hospital, and she has worked every Christmas and every Easter and every public holiday, that's if I haven't done it. This means you are on standby 365 days of the year. Why on earth would I want that? Money is not everything.

I told her that thanks, but no thanks. It is not worth the stress and effort to run the practice. Maybe some people are thinking that I am mad, and that I can get locums to help me out, and yes I can do that and maybe I might just do that, but if they can't work, then I am still responsible for taking up the slack. Do I really want that in my life?

This little quadrant also made me realize that I didn't like doing my little bit of hospital work at the other hospital that I mentioned at the beginning of the chapter. This is when I made the decision to find someone to take it off my hands and saw it as my 10% charity that I was giving away to someone else.

Chapter 11
Breathing

After my car accident and breaking of my ribs, I found it rather painful to breathe. I automatically breathed shallowly and in the upper part of my ribs. I have seen this often in my patients. If they have pneumonia, and it is sore to cough or even breathe then they breathe in their upper lungs. Often this results in a feeling that you just can't get enough air into your lungs. If you test the saturation of your blood, it may be normal, but you feel as if your chest is just not expanding enough to get enough oxygen in.

This is also what happened after my anaesthetic. I had this feeling that I had to sit upright as lying down resulted in my struggling to get air in. My theory is that I had too much fluid in my body and that it was compressing on my lungs which was resulting in this feeling. I have seen this several times in my patients who have heart problems or fluid on their lungs. Some have normal saturation levels and others have low saturation levels.

You may have noticed this in yourself when you are sick and have sinus or lung infections that you can't lay flat as it is just too hard to breathe and makes you feel uncomfortable. This prevents you from sleeping properly. You will have propped yourself up automatically which aids the body in breathing as you have less pressure on your chest in the upright position, but you may not be very comfortable in this position.

I treat little babies with pneumonias and other chest conditions and some struggle to breathe and they are given oxygen to help them feel better. During my treatments I will notice that if I tip them on their tummies to help drain their lungs, they will actually turn blue as they are really struggling to get the air in. They cry uncontrollably as they feel claustrophobic and can't tell you any other way. The pressure of lying on your stomach is just too much and tipping yourself upside down is detrimental. In these conditions I will then treat them more level and not turn them onto their tummies as the chest is just too tight. In these circumstances we use Shortwave to help open the chest up and increase the blood flow to the area. Within 2-3 days of using this, the children are off the oxygen and able to tolerate being placed in the prone position.

Oxygen is vital for life. You need to get enough oxygen in to help the body function properly. In the chart of organ cleaning in a later chapter you see that if you are awake between 3-5am that it could be linked with your lungs as this organ is cleaning house at this time of the day. When you suffer from sinus or chest conditions like asthma, bronchitis and so forth, you will wake up during this time as you are not feeling well.

I have a number of patients who have been struggling with breathing. Some are young and have no apparent medical problems that could cause this and others are older and have many medical problems that can cause this. With the young healthy patients, it could be caused by sinus, or too much sugar, (a bad diet). In my older patients it is often linked with blood clots in the lungs or heart problems again linked with long standing poor health choices. Many of these elderly patients drink coke every day or alcohol in excess; this is detrimental to your health. The medical problems we have as we get older are from life choices we have made over a long period of time and not that quick to reverse and if left too late are not reversible.

I treated a lady who progressively got worse with shortness of breath. She had had a stroke the previous year, but it was a mild stroke and she was on warfarin which was monitored weekly. She was complaining of heaviness in her legs and she was unable to walk far as she would get too tired and her breathing was laboured all the time. She found it easier to purse her lips while breathing. Over a short period of time she got swelling of her feet and I knew that something was not right as her lips were also turning blue. I sent her to the cardiologist and it was discovered that she had blood clots in her lungs from an allergic reaction to warfarin, which had increased her heart chamber drastically and this resulted in the swelling of her feet. They stopped the warfarin immediately and changed her medication and she is now much improved. As it was treated quickly and not left too long, her heart has returned to normal. Remember each person responds differently to medication and what works for one does not always work for the other.

I am treating another gentleman who is also suffering from breathing problems and is often short of breath and struggles to walk due this. He is overweight and has a pacemaker. He is recently retired although he still goes in to the office just to get out of the house as it is his own business. He mentioned that he was drinking quite a lot of alcohol during the day because he was bored and it gave him something to do and he only eats one to two meals per day. I immediately asked him to stop drinking the alcohol as this is very bad for your health. I also advised that he should eat regularly during the day, 4-6 small meals per day to keep his blood sugar levels constant and to help him lose weight. He has already lost 4 kg in the first week and his breathing is better on some days. He still struggles occasionally with shortness of breath and unfortunately this will take a long time to resolve, but he has set the wheel in motion and is eating healthier and drinking healthier and is losing weight. I am hoping that within a short period of time he will be feeling a lot better. Unfortunately as he already has a pacemaker the damage has already been caused so we will not get full recovery.

There are many people who are scared to go to the Doctor and that is not right. We have really good doctors and they are there to help you. You must remember that it is a partnership you are going into and that you need to do your part of improving lifestyle to get better as the medication alone is not going to fix the problem. If you do not like the doctor you are with now, then change and find one that you do like and synergize with. But don't ignore your health, you only have one life.

My tightness of my chest was due to my ribs that were not expanding properly and I had to retrain my ribs and lungs to work properly. When you have pneumonia, or a chest injury or any form of surgery over your chest, you will need to re-educate the movement and have your ribs mobilized. This is done by holding a towel tightly around your lower ribs. You then breathe against the resistance of the towel, so that you can feel where you are supposed to breathe in. As this improves you will get better rib movement and your lungs will be able to expand properly and that feeling of just not enough air will go away.

Another of my patients used to use Iliaden every day as his nose was permanently blocked. Iliaden should only be used for 5 days and then stopped, he said that he used it every 2 hours for years. I was horrified and at once we started using a saline rinse with no medication in it. Many people suffer with Sinus and it can be caused from numerous things. You could be allergic to a range of things or I have a patient who got sinus from staying in a house that had a mould problem. Since this house her sinuses have not improved. Your sinus could further be aggravated by a resistance towards gluten, or that your gut is not working daily and it has caused inflammation in your sinuses. There are many reasons as to why you get sinus.

To improve your sinuses firstly make sure your gut works properly and daily. Then make sure you cut out the factors that you may be allergic to. Such as Gluten or sugars and high gluten index foods. Then you can rinse your sinuses with a saline solution instead of using Iliaden. There are a number of options (a netti pot that looks like Aladdin's lamp), or use sterimar or other saline systems. You rinse half the pot down the one nostril while leaning over a sink letting the water run out the other nostril. If you are too upright, it will run down the back of your throat. Then you turn and rinse the other nostril. When your nostril is blocked then the saline will drip out very slowly or not at all. You then sniff it up and spit it out, this helps open the nostril. After blowing the nose and repeating this a few times (the rinsing), it may run out the other nostril.

My patient who was using Iliaden found that after two days of doing this he could reduce the Iliaden to twice a day. After a week he was able to use it only once a day and after two weeks he could stop the Iliaden. During this cleanse you need to ensure the gut lining is repaired and this is done by firstly eating healthy foods as mentioned in the food chapter. Then you need to repair the gut lining by using special herbs which reduce inflammation such as turmeric and ginger. There are neutraceuticals out there that you can purchase that have a combination of herbs that improve gut lining and depending on your symptoms would depend on the product you would use. I find good neutraceutical companies have a good range that is very good at improving your health and I have seen amazing results in my patients and myself.

If your gut is not working at all, you need to make sure you get neutraceuticals to help you get it moving. Good neutraceutical companies will have good products that can help with this.

A few tips I discovered while working with the kids and having my own, is that when they start getting sick then their hair at the back of their heads gets all tangled and looks like a birds nest. With this they get dry cracked lips and when I look in their ears I can see a build-up of yellow sticky wax. The ear with the bigger build-up is the side that is more blocked as the nose and the ears are connected by a small tube. This is an indication that their noses are blocked and they are breathing through their mouths. This makes the lips dry and cracked. Sinus causes the blocked nose and a chronic sinus will make you snore when you are asleep. Many parents', whose children suffer from chronic sinus, comment on the fact that their child snores. When the birds nest appears it is not long before they will get fever. This birds nest is also an indication that the immune system is compromised as you hair should be soft and silky.

If left untreated and the diet is not altered, then the sinus can cause the tonsils to become inflamed as the secretions are constantly dripping on the tonsils. It can also drip down into the lungs causing tightness of the chest and pneumonia or bronchiolitis. When we start administering antibiotics which at this stage is the only way to treat the illness, then the antibiotics will eradicate the entire good gut flora which causes the leaky gut or other gut issues which will result in a low immune system and the problems just get worse. That is why it is so important to take probiotics when you are taking antibiotics. It is also important to take them for a while after you have taken the antibiotics as one course of antibiotics kills the gut flora for up to a year. If you are not eating healthy foods then you will not replace these gut flora and your health will deteriorate and you will be susceptible to other illnesses (allergies and the like).

A lot of information has been given just on your breathing and sinuses and if you are a bit confused, then start with a really good probiotic, preferably one that has to live in a fridge. This will improve gut function and decrease inflammation.

You are able to measure your breathing using a peak flow meter. This is a good means of determining how effective your lungs are working and you can use this measurement to monitor improvement depending on your intervention. You can also use this to see which intervention works the best or if there is any medication which is affecting your breathing. You can also compare where you should be according to your height and age.

Peak Expiratory Flow Rates

Peak Expiratory Flow Rates

child and adolescent female: 6 - 20 years of age

Height (in)	42	46	50	54	57	60	64	68	72
Age: 6	134	164	193	223	245	268	297	327	357
8	153	182	212	242	264	287	316	346	376
10	171	201	231	261	283	305	335	365	395
12	190	220	250	280	302	324	354	384	414
14	209	239	269	298	321	343	373	403	432
16	228	258	288	318	340	362	392	421	451
18	247	277	306	336	358	381	411	440	470
20	266	295	325	355	377	400	429	459	489

child and adolescent male: 6 - 25 years of age

Height (in)	44	48	52	56	60	64	68	72	76
Age: 6	99	146	194	241	289	336	384	431	479
8	119	166	214	261	309	356	404	451	499
10	139	186	234	281	329	376	424	471	519
12	159	206	254	301	349	396	444	491	539
14	178	226	274	321	369	416	464	511	559
16	198	246	293	341	389	436	484	531	579
18	218	266	313	361	408	456	503	551	599
20	238	286	333	381	428	476	523	571	618
22	258	306	353	401	448	496	543	591	638
24	278	326	373	421	468	516	563	611	658
25	288	336	383	431	478	526	573	621	668

adult female: 20 - 80 years of age

Height (in)	58	60	62	64	66	68	70
Age: 20	357	372	387	402	417	432	446
25	350	365	379	394	409	424	439
30	342	357	372	387	402	417	431
35	335	350	364	379	394	409	424
40	327	342	357	372	387	402	416
45	320	335	349	364	379	394	409
50	312	327	342	357	372	387	401
55	308	320	334	349	364	379	394
60	297	312	327	342	357	372	386
65	290	305	319	334	349	364	379
70	282	297	312	327	342	357	371
75	275	290	304	319	334	349	364
80	267	282	297	312	327	342	356

adult male: 25 - 80 years of age

Height (in)	63	65	67	69	71	73	75	77
Age: 24	492	520	549	578	606	635	664	692
30	481	510	538	567	596	624	653	682
35	471	499	528	557	585	614	643	671
40	460	489	517	546	575	603	632	661
45	450	478	507	536	564	593	622	650
50	439	468	496	525	554	582	611	640
55	429	457	486	515	543	572	601	629
60	418	447	475	504	533	561	590	619
65	408	436	465	494	522	551	580	608
70	397	426	454	483	512	540	569	598
75	387	405	444	473	501	530	559	587
80	376	405	433	462	491	519	548	577

http://www.sh.lsuhsc.edu/fammed/OutpatientManual/PeakFlowTables.htm

Chapter 12
The importance of water

Water is very important for our wellbeing. Our body is made up of about 70% water and our brain 85% water, it is vital to drink the correct amount and quality of water. By drinking the correct amount of water we can improve our health, fitness and even our appearance, by making our skin smoother, softer, more supple with a glowing healthy look. Water acts as a shock absorber in our joints and organs and lubricates our joints. It flushes the kidneys of toxins as well as improves kidney function. It balances electrolytes in our body helping to manage our blood pressure. It can improve energy levels, increase physical and mental performance and even help us lose weight. It also allows proper digestion and helps keep us more alkaline. I am sure you did not realize how many things water actually does for us.

The amount of water one should be drinking each day depends on how much you weigh. If you weigh 60kg then 2 Litres is sufficient. The more you weigh the more you should drink, this is worked out as your weight in Kg multiplied by 0.033L. This amount of water also varies depending on the weather, so the hotter the weather and the more you sweat the more water you should be drinking. It is recommended that 500ml of water is added per 30min of moderate exercise. If you drink water 15 minutes before you eat, you will improve the digestion of your food, but if you drink during your meal you decrease the acid in your stomach decreasing your digestion.

If you are thirsty, then you are already 10% dehydrated. The less you drink the more you will be constipated and your brain will be less active causing poor concentration. You will feel tired and your heart will have to work harder to circulate your blood, increasing your blood pressure.

You can drink too much water and I have had several patients who inform me they are drinking 3-5 litres per day. These patients' tell me that they are constantly thirsty which is why they are drinking so much water. An intense thirst can mean that your body is heading towards becoming a diabetic or is already a diabetic or that your omega 3 levels are too low. These are all symptoms one needs to be aware of. When your thirst is under control and you are drinking your correct amount of water per day without having this thirst, then you are improving your body functioning. I heard on the radio a story of a challenge that was put out to the audience and the person who drank the most amount of water over a two day period would win a huge prize. A male student took on the challenge and drank so much water that he died. This was obviously not the intention of the radio presenter and he did not know that if you drank too much water that you could die.

Many people are of the opinion that drinking tap water is still okay and that it is a waste of money to buy filtered water or bottled water. Personally since I have been studying further and seen what tap water contains I am scared to drink tap water and would rather not drink anything than drink tap water. Our tap water and other sources of water can be polluted by the lead in the pipes, from the microbiological growth inside the pipeline or tank and rusting pipes or holding tanks and chloride from the PVC pipes. The Chlorination process that happens in the municipal water supplies can cause chloroform which is a toxin to our bodies. Some times when I am in the shower I can actually smell the chlorine and am grateful that I don't have to drink it. I have seen experiments where tap water is taken and two electrodes placed in the water and a current sent through the electrodes. After a short current the water turns brown at the top and when tested it is shown to be faeces drifting in the water.

I read the book set *"The secret life of water ", "The hidden messages of water" and "The True power of water" by Masaru Emoto*. In these books he talks about water being a living entity that can read our thoughts. He would take pictures of water from all different sources on a microscopic level showing the different crystal formation. In sludgy water there would be no crystal formation, but when he prayed over the water and told the water that he was grateful for the water and retook the pictures, they formed the most beautiful crystals. Each picture of water molecules had a totally different form and shape of crystal.

Education is power and firstly knowing that my water was not of the best quality, I decided to invest in a water purification system. There are many out there and often one is confused as to which is the best and if the water tastes nice then it must be good. I attended several lectures where they would talk about the differences between the different water purification systems and there is one that came out tops.

I have attached the water purification comparison chart and it indicates that the E-spring water purification is one of the top water purification systems available in our own homes and at an affordable price. Since investing in my own E-Spring I find that I am unable to drink tap water or other forms of water elsewhere. I make sure that I carry my bottles around town with my own water in them, to avoid drinking tap water. It has been shown that certain plastic bottles leak chemicals into your water when they get hot. The studies have indicated that this causes disease as our bodies cannot process these toxins. We need to use bottles that have been specifically made to prevent this from happening as the plastic is of a higher quality. Alternatively you can use glass bottles. I have purchased bottles that will not leak chemicals into my water when it does get hot as there is no point in having good water when you have bad bottles to hold it.

There is a Doctor in the Cape who specializes in treating patients suffering from cancer. She recommends an E-spring as one of the first items they must purchase when working towards improving their health. Your body is made up of so much water, that it is very important to ensure you are giving your body the best opportunity possible to heal.

Not only are we susceptible to illness from drinking chlorinated water, so are our animals and our plants. I use my water to fill the animals drinking bowls and I use it to wash my fruit and vegetables and boil water for coffee. My plants outside get rainwater collected from our gutters into big drums and occasionally tap water when the drums are empty.

Comparisons With Other Water Treatment Technologies

Water Treatment Technology Options	Technology Overview	Technology Improves			Technology Reduces			
		Taste	Smell	Clarity	Contaminating particles	Organic compounds	Chlorine by-products	Cysts
Water Treatment System with activated carbon block filter & UV lamp	Activated carbon block adsorbs up to 140 types of contaminants. UV light removes up to 99.99% of waterborne bacteria and viruses.	★	★	★	★	★	★	★
Boiling	Does not remove contaminating particles, organic or inorganic compounds in water. May release volatile organic compounds into the air. Time consuming and inconvenient.	×	●	×	×	●	● ~~×~~	★
Reverse osmosis	Slow and inefficient. 80-90% of water wastage. Needs high pressure. May remove beneficial minerals in water. Limited volume.	● ~~★~~	● ~~★~~	★	★	●	●	★
Alkaline water (with calcium)	No evidence that this method could improve water quality. Does not remove contaminating particles, organic or inorganic compound, bacteria or viruses.	×	×	×	×	×	×	×
Activated carbon particulate	Most of them do not remove waterborne contaminants, organic or inorganic compound or bacteria/viruses. A fixed flow path is most likely to form inside the filter, resulting in untreated effluent.	★	★	●	●	●	●	×
Water filtration bottle or pitcher type	Most of them do not remove organic or inorganic contaminants. The filter treats only a limited amount of water. Filter needs regular replacement.	★	★	★	●	●	●	●
Bottled water	Quality varies with each brand and batch. Some do not not remove volatile organic compound or inorganic contaminants. Inconvenient and costly.	●	●	●	●	●	●	●
Hollow fibre	Effectively removes contaminating particles and bacteria in the short term, but barely works on viruses or organic contaminants. Needs chlorine to control bacteria growth.	●	●	★	★	×	×	★

22 eSpring reference guide

The following chart shows that many of these common treatment methods have the potential for improving water quality. But notice that no single technology or method addresses all the contaminants that may be present in your water. Nor do they all adequately address the issues of efficiency as determined by the amount of water that can be provided in a reasonable time or ongoing maintenance costs. By comparison, the combined carbon filter with ultraviolet light technology of the eSpring Water Treament System is far superior, illustrating a full spectrum of capabilities.

★ *Effective* ● *May Be Effective* × *Not Effective* **N/A** *Not Applicable*

			Benefits						
Inorganic compounds	**Bacteria**	**Viruses**	**Retains beneficial minerals**	**Fast filtration**	**Any volume on demand**	**Low treated cost**	**Replacement lasts 1 year**	**Monitoring systems**	**Easy installation**
●	★	★	★	★	★	★	★	★	★
×	★	★	★	×	×	★	N/A	N/A	N/A
★	●	●	×	×	×	●	●	●	●
×	×	×	★	●	★	★	●	●	★
×	×	×	★	★	★	★	●	●	●
●	×	×	●	×	×	×	×	●	★
●	●	●	●	●	×	×	N/A	N/A	N/A
×	●	●	★	●	★	●	●	●	●

Chapter 13
You are what you eat

When I was in the UK I was treating a very overweight lady for lower back pain. She used to walk with a pram because she did not have enough strength to stand up straight. She had been sent to a dietician for advice and had been following her suggestions religiously. However, what she had not been told was that she could not eat apple pie for pudding every night. She would tell me what she ate for breakfast, lunch and supper and when I asked her if there was anything else she put in her mouth in the form of cold drinks or puddings, this apple pie crept up into the equation. When I told her that it was not good to eat apple pie on a daily basis as she literally looked like an apple, she told me that her mom had given it to them every day and she thought that it was the right thing to do.

Many of my patients tell me that their mom and brothers also look the way they do or have the same problem they have and that it must be genetic. However it is also what one is brought up with and the foods we eat. We have a tendency to cook the same way our mothers did and thus we duplicate it in our homes and wonder why we have the same problems as our parents. So it is not only genetic but environmental too. You have a predisposition for getting a certain disease according to your genetic makeup, but if you eat incorrectly you will activate these genes and get the disease. If you eat correctly you can keep these genes dormant and have good health.

There is this book I read that was talking about irritable bowel and other bowel problems. *"Follow your gut" by Rob Knight.* In this book they mentioned that when a mother gives birth to her baby naturally, the baby moves through the birth canal and gets covered with all her bacteria she has in her body, so if the mom suffers from bad bowel movements and problems, then so will the child because it is governed by your gut flora. The only way to fix this is to take a good probiotic and improve your colony in your gut, which will improve your bowel movements and improve a lot of your problems. It was also stated that if you do have bowel problems that this will cause inflammation in the body and this in turn causes all kinds of other medical problems, from sinus, asthma, arthritis, diabetes depression and many other diseases. So it is essential to ensure that you eat the right foods and have the right flora in your gut, so that it can function optimally.

I did a little experiment at home myself. Each night I had a craving for something sweet. I would eat a rusk with Milo or I would eat a chocolate or some days some chips (crisps). It took 5 weeks for me to suddenly expand around my waste and buttock and look a little frumpy. Now to turn this the other way round was a night mare and takes way longer than 5 weeks to lose what you gained, this of course is just by not eating the rubbish. Sometimes one would need to implement a healthy eating program to lose this excess weight if you are not already eating healthily.

When I was telling my patients about this, the one lady had an epiphany. She suddenly realized why she had gained 10kg in her matric year. She told me her story of how each day in matric she and her friend would buy a chocolate and share it. She said that if she had known it would have such an adverse effect on her, she would never have done it. But since then she has not been able to lose the 10kg and as she gets older, she just adds on another few Kgs and had no idea as to why it was happening. Since then she has modified her diet and cut out all the sugar and refined carbohydrates and has since lost most of the weight.

As one gets older it is much harder to keep slim. You are not nearly as active as you were at school; you don't have your sport every afternoon unless you have made a special effort to ensure you are still exercising on a regular basis. You have more stress and more responsibilities and find that there is no such thing as a balance between resting, play hard and work hard. It is mostly just work, work, work and running kids around and cook dinner, or get takeaways, because you are too tired to cook and don't have the inclination to cook or your cooking is revolting.

When I went to the UK the first time round, I thought it was heaven when I walked into the shops and saw buy one get one free. So I would buy lasagne for each night of the week as it was my favourite dinner. As I was no longer at home and I was an adult, I could chose when I ate sweets and which sweets I could eat. I would buy fruit pastels and have them at the ready. They also had frozen cakes, of course my favourite ones and each week I would buy a different one, they had lemon meringue, cheese cake and Pavlova. Since you could not refreeze the cakes, it would mean that I would have to eat the whole cake on my own and you can't leave it too long as it would go off, so I would eat the cake in about 3-4 days all by myself. I would wake up in the morning and eat some fruit pastels that were lying on my bedside table. Then I would have yogurt and muesli for breakfast. I would pack my lunch with a cheese and salami bread roll with a bunch of grapes. Then I would come home and eat a slice of cake and then I would have my lasagne with corn. I ate this every single day for about 3 months. When things coming out the other side started looking like what went in, I started wondering if it was such a good idea to continue to eat it every day.

At this stage as I had not learnt anything about nutrition and I thought I was eating healthily. Of course the cake and sweets were not really considered a problem, in my mind, so surely I did not need to stop taking them. What happened was that I gained so much weight; I went from a size 8 to a size 14 in 8 months. I ripped my pants during the one day at work, much to my horror.

I returned to South Africa and the buy one get one free special was no longer available and I had moved back home with my folks, so I was eating normal food again and a variety. I lost all my weight again and felt good being slim again.

A few years later I went back to the UK. I once again started gaining my weight and got a blocked nose. It got to a point where I started getting heart palpitations and if I had an afternoon nap, my eyelid would swell. And yet I still did not think that it could be my food. My body was sore and getting worse, I was getting dead legs and cramping of any muscle if I remotely did a little bit of exercise. I would also snore myself awake and every Friday night I would suffer from diarrhoea, because of the pizza I ate. That took me a year to discovery it was the pizza and only after I had attended the course.

It was during this time when I went on the Chan Gunn course and was exposed to the idea of metabolic insufficiencies, that I started realizing that diet could influence my body. It also explained all the weird symptoms that the Dr could not give me a pill for. This was when I went on the Nutrition and lifestyle course with Paul Check and was taught the importance of eating correctly.

After the course I remember sitting in the kitchen and wondering what to eat. I wanted to make an egg, but I could not eat the bread, so how do you have egg on toast when you can't eat the toast? And what do you have for lunch if you can't have a sandwich? I was confused and it took me about 4 months to understand what it was that I could eat and how to make salads and healthy options of lunch and supper and breakfast. I also found the importance of eating snacks to keep your blood sugar levels normal. I started asking my patients what they were eating and their diets were as bad as my own was. They too could not believe that their diet could influence them as much as it does. I am still amazed at what diet can do for you.

So I read the "*The metabolic typing diet*" by William Wolcott and I was amazed at how quickly people felt better. Within a week your energy levels are improved and within two weeks you feel much better from what you felt like. The unfortunate thing is that you still can't get everything from your diet. The reason for this is that food is far less nutritious than it was 50years ago. Research shows that the vitamins and minerals you got from one lettuce head 50 years ago, is equivalent to 20 lettuce heads now. This means that you will never get what your body needs in your meals. So we now need to add supplementation to the equation. It has been shown that one would need a minimum of a multivitamin and an omega 3 supplement. The problem is that you can't just buy any one off the shelf as if it is synthetic and not organic and natural, then you can actually cause more medical problems than not taking one at all.

I made sure that I was taking everything that I needed, both supplements and eating. I was eating correctly for 10 years before I harvested my eggs. This drain to my system was so severe that my normal vitamin and diet regime was no longer enough to support my body and I needed to get advanced neutraceuticals to improve the imbalance in my body. I started getting cravings that had been under control for a long time. I had the itchy nose and itchy eyes and blocked nose again and clicking nose and the list goes on. I knew that my diet was important and I was still trying to eat most of the time a good nutritious meal, but my energy levels were so low that it was getting hard to continue making the healthy meals and then I fell off the wagon into the ditch. The neutraceuticals were very helpful in getting me back on track.

I mentioned the importance of good probiotics in your gut, but the reason for this is huge. Your gut must work on a daily basis and it must be a big brown one. Yes it's a bit graphic, but the colour and stench is all indicative of how healthy you are. If you are not dumping the load daily, then you are holding toxins back in your body which cause inflammation throughout the body activating those genes and switching on the diseases.

So you need to eliminate items out of your diet that are causing your gut to become permeable. This includes sugar and refined carbohydrates. There are also certain foods that some people are more allergic to than others and these can also be eliminated for a short period of time to ensure you are not one of the people who do have an allergy towards them.

Through attending multiple courses I have learnt that it is vitally important to eat a range of different foods. So don't eat lasagne every day and the same breakfast every day and the same lunch every day. You need to vary your breakfast and lunch and supper. The more you vary the foods going in, the more you vary the enzymes that are digesting the food. You also get a larger range of vitamins and minerals entering your body which helps to keep all the little irritating things at bay that you don't go to the Doctor for.

I learnt about the 4 day rotation diet through the check institute and I have been using this extensively. What does this mean?

Over 4 days you will eat 4 different items of proteins for dinner. You are only allowed to eat this protein again within a 24 hour period and then not again for 4 days. This avoids an increased sensitivity towards the food.

As an example you would eat chicken for supper on the first day and make double so you can eat it for lunch the next day. The second day you would eat fish and have tuna for lunch the day after (I could not eat left over fish the next day), on day 3 you would eat lamb and repeat again for lunch and then on day four you would eat game or pork. Now we mentioned that pork and beef was on the elimination list, due to the fact that some people can be hyper allergic to them, so if you are allergic or you are doing the elimination section then the pork and beef would not be eaten. Also if you are a vegetarian then of course that would be eliminated too, but make sure you are getting enough proteins in your diet as this is very important for the building blocks in your body and you can get very ill if you do not get enough proteins in.

I had a patient who was an avid runner and competed in all the long distance marathons. When she came to me she was experiencing severe pains in her legs. Her pains were so severe that she was unable to even jog around the block and had stopped all training. It turned out that she was a vegetarian and because she was training so hard, her body was taking the vitamins and minerals out of her muscles just to function normally, but when there are no more nutrients to take, then the muscles become painful and you are unable to continue with your normal regime. So we had to increase her protein intake even if it is in the form of plants and added protein powders into all her meals.

I have also learnt the importance of eating the green leafy vegetables. The green leave vegetables are the most important part of reverting your DNA back to the original state, switching off those activated genes. You should have a range of leafy greens for lunch and supper. These improve your fibre content and improve weight loss. Fibre is any fruit or vegetable.

The importance of the different colours of vegetables for your diet, go as follows:

Red: for prostate health and cell health: cranberries, watermelon, pink grapefruit, guava, pomegranate, radishes, raspberries, strawberries, cherries, tomatoes, red apples.

Orange and yellow: eye health, healthy immune function, maintains skin hydration, healthy growth and development: oranges, carrots, apricots, sweet potatoes, tangerines, squash, papaya, corn, pineapples, lemons, granadillas.

Green: Cell health, support arterial function, lung health, maintains healthy liver function: kale, collard greens, spinach, green peppers, watercress, lettuce, Zucchini, broccoli, Brussel sprouts, green beans, soybeans, green tea.

Blue and purple: cognitive health, heart health, support arterial function, and antioxidant protection: Figs, grapes, blueberries, mulberries, red cabbage, black currents, eggplant, purple sweet potatoes, black beans, plums, beets, blackberries.

White: Maintain healthy bones, circulatory health, support arterial function: Turnips, onions, mushrooms, horseradish, white kidney beans, parsnips, garlic, cauliflower, black eyed peas, pears.

One would need to get a range of different colours in each day to ensure you are getting the correct vitamins and minerals to support these functions. I find that if you cut them up small and put them all in the salad and then drizzle a little balsamic vinegar or apple cider vinegar over the top, then the items that you don't like to eat all taste the same (vinegar) and it goes down the hatch quite easily. Then there are none of the issues with the fact that you don't like eating them because they don't taste nice. It's a different thing if you are allergic to them. Please ensure you are not eating things you are allergic to!

Now you have eliminated the items that can give you allergic reactions, you are eating salads like a little buck. You are eating regularly, at least breakfast, lunch and supper. Now we need to add the little snacks in between. It is advised that one should not go without food for more than 3 hours. This slows your metabolism down and causes problems with the blood sugar levels. You need a healthy snack between breakfast and lunch and lunch and supper and if you struggle to sleep then a nice little snack before going to bed. The regulation of your blood sugar levels will prevent you getting mood swings. It will keep your energy levels constant and it will keep you healthy. You can't run a car with no petrol, so you must remember that you can't run your body without food either, this is your petrol.

When I came back from the UK, I was treating this young man who had just started working. He was working long hours and was complaining of weakness and fatigue and poor concentration. He was extremely tall and thin and when I asked him to do some simple movements, he had poor body control and was unable to do these movements. When I asked him about his diet he reported that he was drinking 36 cups of coffee a day to keep him going. He did not eat breakfast or lunch and only had two minute noodles for supper. He was constantly nauseous and was really not feeling good.

I immediately worked on his diet and he started eating a healthy lunch and supper. He cut his coffee down to a maximum of three per day. He was able to do his exercises much better and felt a lot better. He still reported feeling nauseous in the morning when he got up. This nausea only left at 12h00. When I asked him the time he ate his first meal of the day, he stated that it was at 11am. When I pointed out that the nausea went away at 12h00 which was an hour after he ate and that it would be a good idea to eat breakfast to eliminate the nausea he was a little surprised. Breakfast is the breaking of the fast from the nights' sleep, which is what breakfast means. The type of breakfast you eat will set your entire day.

If you eat a nice healthy substantial breakfast, it will sustain you throughout the day and make you feel awake, mentally ready and eager for anything that comes your way. If you do not eat breakfast, you will feel nauseous, tired, irritated, and anxious or run down. If you eat an unhealthy breakfast it can bloat you and make you feel tired, irritated, anxious and worried and unwell. Your food is very important and you must ensure you eat regularly.

But this goes for any meal. I had a gentleman patient who had his own company and he mentioned to me that every afternoon his employees had to stay clear of him as he would be in a really bad mood. When I asked him what he was eating for lunch, he would state that it was usually a sandwich or a noodle salad. When I mentioned that it may be the starch that was affecting him, and I suggested that he have a salad instead, it made a huge difference. Just cutting out the refined starch in the form of white bread and the noodles, made him feel much better and calmer.

I find that if I am feeling a bit tired, if I snack on a salad with a bit of protein, then my energy is boosted again and I can continue with what I need to do. If however, I have a toasted chicken sandwich, then my energy tanks even more and I feel quite irritated and want to sleep.

It is nice to eat sweets and chips and burgers and pizza, I don't deny it, but the fact that they drain your energy and make you feel awful is beyond denial. If you reduce the amount of times you eat fast foods and unhealthy snacks and sweets, then your body is able to handle it on a much better scale. It is suggested that you have takeaways only once a month or less. What I do is I say to my son, that we have junk Fridays. So we get a take away on a Friday or we can have a sweet. If Vincent has a sporting event on the Saturday then we have it on the Saturday night instead, so that his energy is not low for the event. What I have found though is that when we do get the take away, they don't taste as nice as they used to and they really don't make us feel that good, and the desire to eat them has reduced substantially.

I like to think of it as the 90/10 rule. 90% of the time you stick to the path and 10% of the time you can eat a sweet or burger and chips. This makes it about 3 meals per week that you can cheat. When you are eating healthy and you have cut out the unhealthy foods for at least 2 weeks before cheating, you will notice that you feel so bad when you do eat the rubbish food, that you are not going to want to eat it that often and then may only eat it at parties or when you go out as a treat.

One of my patients who followed my suggestions with her family and removed the refined carbohydrates and sugars and only fed her children healthy snacks for school and at home, had amazing results. In one term their marks improved by 10%. This is a significant number; it could be the difference between passing and failing or getting a good mark and getting a distinction. One is able to concentrate much better and sit still for longer, when you are eating the right foods. You don't feel tired and you don't get hungry and you don't get cravings and you can study more in the same amount of time or get more done in the same amount of time.

Another of my patients was diabetic and taking medication for it. His sugar levels were sitting at 9. They should be 5. When I asked him what he was eating he told me that he had Simba chips for breakfast or a pie or bag of peanuts for the protein. He had no actual idea of what to eat or how to go about improving his health. When I discussed the diet plan with him and gave him some ideas, which he followed, his health improved drastically. His sugar went down to a 6 within the first week and to a 4 by the second week.

His energy levels were improved and his concentration was better. It would take a while before he lost his little pot belly tummy, but at least he was on the road to recovery.

Yet another patient was suffering from diabetes and was struggling to walk due to leg and back pain and did not sleep well. He also had a little pot belly and his energy was low. Within a week his sugar had dropped again and by the second week it was almost normal. His energy picked up and his blood pressure improved too. He slept better and his pains in his legs and back went away totally. He lost his little pot belly and was feeling very good. He found that after a few months of eating correctly, when he did cheat and have a piece of cake his sugar levels did not spike like they did in the past. Previously when he ate cake, he would feel really bad and his sugar would spike very high. He was following the 90/10 rule, but as he had lost all his weight and was feeling good, the effect of the 10% was negligent.

If you are feeling bad and you have recently had a meal. You need to think about what it was that you ate, as within one and half hours to two hours your body will respond to the food you have fed it. This is very quick. If you are eating healthily you will feel better after your meal and gradually reverse the negative effects that bad eating has caused. This reminds me of a story I read in the book *"The compound effect"* by Darren Hardy.

The story tells of a man who was seen as very dynamic. He was a manager at his work that was respected by his colleagues and was approachable and fun. He would come home every afternoon and spend quality time with his two boys either playing a sport or rough housing. He would walk around the block every day with his wife and they would discuss the matters of the day and were very close. He never had time for TV and overall was leading a happy balanced life. One Sunday he decided to treat his job well done.

He decided that he enjoyed the baking so much that he would bake every Sunday enough muffins for the week. Each day he would have two muffins for breakfast. This went on for a number of months. Finally towards the end of the year he had gained a lot of weight. He was feeling tired and did not feel up to playing with his sons and had no energy to walk around the block with his wife. He opted to sit in front of the TV and do nothing. Gradually this became the norm of the day and everything that he had been good at before became not only a chore to do, but he was no longer good at it. He was no longer excelling at work and had been called into the office for a stern talking to. He had increased blood pressure and cholesterol and was tired. His relationships both with his wife and kids were taking strain and he was unhappy.

This was all due to the muffins he had decided to eat on a daily basis.

In the book *"The slight edge" by Jeff Olson* he talks about how making a small change in your life can have compounding effects on health, finances and the list goes on. He states that if you monitor two people who take two different options, that within a two year period they will be on opposite sides of the spectrum. So if we take one person who decides to eat healthily and another who has a coke and chips regularly, by the end of the two years the one will be healthy and happy and the other one will be overweight and unhealthy. Often the overweight people then turn around and say to the skinny healthy person "You are so lucky." Sad to say, luck has nothing to do with it. It takes hard work and dedication.

The catch though is it is not the big things that make a difference; it is the little things that you change that make the big difference over time. It is just as easy to choose to eat the burger as it is to eat the chicken salad. It is easy to choose to drink a coke or drink water. The choice is up to you to make, but in the long run, the healthier option is always better.

My son has learnt a lot about healthy eating and knows that certain foods will make him hyperactive and others not. He has noticed that when he looks in the lunchboxes at school, that the children who are naughty and disruptive are always the kids who have junk food in their lunchboxes and many of them have never event tasted a sweet pea. He even has one little girl who begs him to swap his lunch. She will swap him her doughnut for his celery and sweet peas. He has agreed to help her only on a Friday when he knows its junk day. He has enough understanding of what the food does that he has the will power to say no.

He has asked me several times why is it that the other children have such unhealthy foods and that when teacher looks in their lunch boxes she tells them that they have healthy lunchboxes. I have noticed that the school is still teaching the children the old food pyramid and you will still recognize it from your school days as it has not changed in the text books. However, it has changed in the medical field and there are several courses being offered that indicate the food pyramid is actually the other way round

THE HEALTHY EATING PYRAMID

Department of Nutrition, Harvard School of Public Health

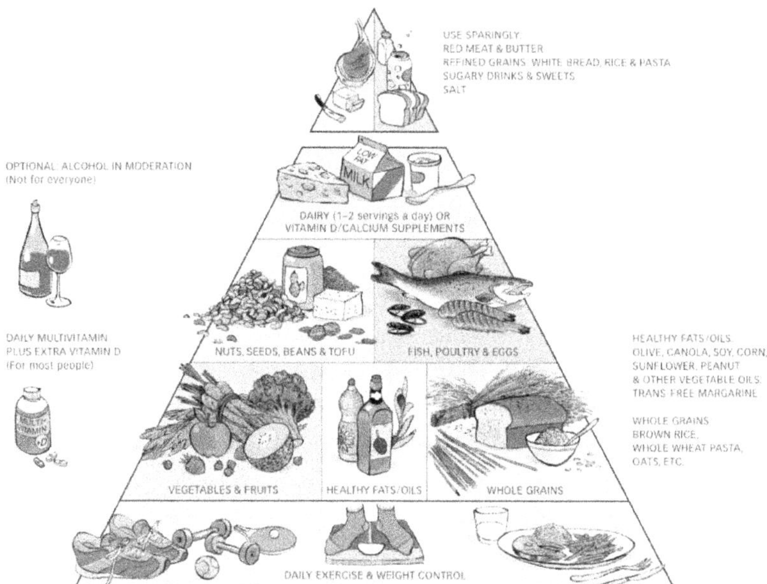

The Healthy Eating Pyramid, adapted from Eat, Drink and Be Healthy, *by Walter C. Willett and Patrick J. Skerrett, Simon and Schuster/Free Press, 2005. Copyright 2008, President and Fellows of Harvard College.*

Bread and refined starch are at the top of the pyramid and should be consumed very seldom. Unfortunately as the old food pyramid is still being taught in all the schools, it is going to be a slow process of education starting with those that are sick and desperate and others who are interested in maintaining a healthy lifestyle. Those that fall in the cracks are the majority and the ones that are going to suffer the most.

Just out of interest as to how the food pyramid came about. During the world wars, the government would ensure that the meat would go to the fighting men in the wars. Thus meat sold in the home towns became very expensive and unaffordable for the women and children staying behind. They needed to make a plan and started making bread to fill the tummies. When the men returned years later this had become the norm of what was given for food and thus they too began eating bread. This is why the food pyramid states that bread needs to be the biggest part of our daily intake of food. Allergies were unheard prior to 1819. During this year it became known as an epidemic just a few years after the war when all the people had been eating unhealthy breads.

Unfortunately high starch and sugary foods cause leaky gut and inflammation throughout the body. This is why we have the better options of Low GI and gluten free breads available in the shops and lately the addition of gluten free pizza bases and whole wheat breads.

If you want to test how good your gut is working and whether it is breaking down the food correctly or absorbing it correctly you can test it by monitoring your elimination time. This is done by eating corn or beetroot. I prefer the corn as it is easier to see. You take note of the day and time that you eat the corn. You then wait for it to exit the other side. If it is within 24-48 hours then you have a good colon transit time. If it is shorter, then you are not digesting your food properly and you can look into methods to improve this. If it is longer, then you are reabsorbing the toxins and giving the parasites more time to feed on the food, making your body ill and toxic.

I do hope that you have received some insight as to how you should be eating in this chapter and work slowly towards changing the way you eat to ensure you improve your quality of life. As mentioned before, food has the biggest ability to improve your quality of life, but you have to have the mental will power to stay the course.

Chapter 14
Exercising

After my car accident I attended physio treatments where she would do Pilates exercises with me. They helped strengthen my body and were quite effective. If combined with the needling they are potent. While in the UK, I went on courses which led me to be able to be an instructor in Pilates. We focused on doing modified Pilates as most of the people we work with are in such pain, that they are unable to do the Pilates classes that are offered at the local gym. So we use these modified exercises to build them up to a point where they are then able to join the gym and take it further.

Pilates was actually created by a gentleman called Joseph Pilates. He was held captive during the war in the concentration camps and was determined that he would survive. As he was generally a sickly person and had poor muscle strength, he decided that the only way he was going to survive was if he got his body into tip top shape. He started working with what he had available in the camps. Mostly Pilates uses your own body weight as resistance and as there were beds with springs, there are some exercises that you do using a reformer, which is a bed with springs that you do the exercises on. Now we use exercise balls and foam rollers to make the Pilates exercises more difficult, and different, but you don't need them when you get started. You don't even have to lie on the floor as you can start on your bed.

The one thing that you must be aware of is that pain causes a reduction in muscle strength. Within 48 hours of an injury taking place the muscles will be weaker and this weakness in turn causes more pain. It is a progressive cycle and gets worse without intervention. My chronic pain patients are often in too much pain to even consider any form of exercise. Those that have tried Pilates at the gym often find a substantial increase in their pain and become afraid of all forms of exercise. It is essential to get your body stronger if you want to get rid of the pain.

Let me give you an example. Many years ago while working in the UK, I was called into a cubicle by one of my junior Physios who had this patient whom they had no idea what to do with. He was a gentleman in his thirties who had such severe back pain he was walking with two crutches. His MRI scan was clear and the Doctor said there was nothing wrong with him. He was on many pain pills, but none of them were helping. He was complaining of pain in his back and down his legs and when he walked I was shocked to see his upper half of his body sheering from side to side on his lower half of his body. I knew that he had severe weakness and that nothing we did manually would help the pain, we had to strengthen the area up, but cycling or walking or any other form of exercise made his pain worse. I recommended that he start modified Pilates exercises with only one exercise per day. We started with the pelvic floor exercises and tried to add it to the leg slide exercise. As he started moving his leg he experienced pins and needles down his leg as he had no core control at all.

In Pilates, you are not supposed to feel an increase in pain and you are not to continue with the exercises if you get shaking, as this is an indication that the muscle has fatigued and other muscles take over the action to compensate. This is not conducive to getting better. As he was experiencing pins and needles down his legs doing the modified exercises, I had to improvise and modify the modified exercises. He agreed to do the pelvic floor exercises for two weeks, as the basis for core strengthening. The catch was that he had to do them every two hours. Little but often!

Pelvic floor stimulation in simple language is when you have to tighten your anus. By focusing on this area you will automatically contract your pelvic floor muscle which is the part in front of your anus. Do not tighten your buttocks or your legs, but your anus only. After two weeks of doing this we tried the leg slide again, he was able to slide his leg half way before he experienced pain and pins and needles in his legs. So we did half a leg slide with the anus tightening exercises for another two weeks. Only after these 2 weeks was he able to do a full leg slide. We then tried to add the bridging exercise and gradually kept adding the exercises one by one modifying each one as we went. It took us 6 months, but we were able to get him walking without his crutches and we were able to get him to stop taking his pain medication as he no longer had pain. He was also healthy enough and strong enough to return to work. This simple form of exercise changed his life and he was over the moon. He continued with his exercises and I am sure he is still doing them, but he has a normal functioning life now.

I had another elderly lady who had undergone surgery to remove her bowels in exchange for a colonoscopy bag. Since the surgery she was complaining of left leg pain and when she came to see me she was unable to straighten her leg. She also had a care taker who had to stay with her 24/7 as she was unable to lift her buttocks for a bed pan. She was unable to turn herself in her bed; she was unable to walk and needed someone else to do everything for her. As she was unable to do the exercises as she was just too weak, I had to modify the modified exercises, but told her that she needed to do the exercises every 2 hours.

Remember to only do the exercises until you experience pain or shaking, then you stop, but if you repeat it every two hours, you will get huge improvement in a short period of time. She worked at it religiously, only able to do about 2 repetitions in the beginning. But after two weeks, she was able to turn in bed, lift her buttocks all the way up onto her shoulders. She was able to sit over the edge of the bed on her own and she was able to walk with a Zimmer frame. Two weeks further along, she was walking with a walking stick and her pain was gone in her leg and she no longer needed the care taker.

For years later she used to attend the exercise classes I gave at the old age home. She used to motivate everyone to come to class as she was keen to keep herself as mobile as possible for as long as possible. She had no pain and was keen to try new exercises to help her further. She told me that considering she was stuck in the bed and was not able to do anything anyway, that she might as well do her exercises as it was something to do. Well that something got her walking again and she was forever grateful.

There was yet another patient I had who was so weak in his shoulders that he was unable to take his shirt off without bending forward to lift the arms. He used gravity to lift the arms and initially I did not realize what he was doing as it was so natural for him to do it that way, until I asked him what he was doing. He was under the care of a rheumatologist and had been admitted into hospital for infiltration. I saw him to give him advice on his lifestyle and diet as well as give him Pilate's exercises to strengthen him up. When I saw this we had to modify the modified exercises and he had to work hard at getting his arm to lift again. He did win and that arm could lift in standing again, but again about 6 months to get there.

If you exercise regularly and still don't get benefit, the relevant muscle may be torn and surgery may be the only answer. I was in the advice clinic in the UK and we had a referral of a young guy to the physio department for improvement of shoulder range of movement. The history indicated that his shoulder muscle was torn off and that surgery was needed. The special test I did confirmed it to be off and we referred him to surgery. Sonar of your shoulder or an MRI scan will show clearly if the muscle is off or not. There are also special tests that confirm this. It is worth going to see an orthopaedic surgeon to help you resolve this matter, if conservative treatment has not helped. They will know what to do and you will get physio after to ensure you get full range again.

If I see a flicker of muscle working then then it is likely that one can coax it to do more. Obviously if there is nothing then one can't get it to work, but I remember this gentleman who had had a brachial plexus injury. The brachial plexus is a large nerve that comes out the neck and then splits up into the three main nerves that run down the arm and make the arm work and feel and do everything. If it is cut, then it will never work again, if it is compressed or pulled, then we can try coaxing it to work again but there needs to be some form of a flicker in the muscles. In his case his nerve had not been severed. He was unable to lift his arm or perform any other tasks, but there was a flicker in the fingers.

He had no elbow function, no wrist function and only slight twitching of his fingers. I am grateful that we had physio assistants in the UK, as I would recommend which exercises she needed to do with him and the two of them would get moving. After two weeks I would re-evaluate him and advance his exercises and off they would go again. He came three times a week as we used slings to help him exercise and these are not easy to have at home and assistance with the routine is required.

When the arm is too weak to do the exercises on its own, slings are used to hold the arm up and take gravity out of the equation to enable the muscle to work without resistance. In the UK and some rehabilitation clinics here they have grids attached to the ceiling. The slings are hooked into these grids and positioned over the joints in the body. You can retrain the arm or the leg using this method.

This man would have to lie on his side and we would sling his arm at the wrist and at the elbow. He would then swing his arm backwards and forwards activating the muscles in his arm as there was no weight of the arm. This feels really nice and easy. He could move his elbow, his shoulder and his wrist all using this position.

As he strengthened we let him lie on his back and do the same movements. Once he could do this easily he would then try it without the slings with a shortened lever (bent elbow) and then we straighten the elbow and so the progress goes along. It is a slow process and one can become despondent, which is why it is good to have someone motivate you all the way. Our little assistant Nicolle was great like that, she is a bubbly person and if worried would get me to pop my head in to make sure they were doing it right and motivate both of them that everything was on target and progressing perfectly.

He was determined to get his arm better as most of the British are. If you tell them to do an exercise every two hours, they will ask you if they need to wake up during the night to do them as well. They will also do the exercises until they are told otherwise by another physio or the same physio. They will do the exercises till the day they die. Most South Africans will first question why they need to do the exercises. If they remember they may Google the exercise and decide that there is something else better to do. Or mostly they just forget to do the exercise as our lifestyles are too busy.

Those that do the exercise after been told a story of someone else who did it and found that it worked, will reap the benefits. Some have been suffering so long that they are desperate to try anything and then follow the regime to the letter.

This gentleman worked for 6 months three times a week in our gym and did whatever he could at home as well. After 6 months he was able to lift his arm up above his head and he had full range of motion and he was ecstatic. I happened to meet him at a pub a few months down the line and he was having fun with his cricket buddies and was going to join the cricket team again as he was able to use his arm normally again. That is true dedication.

I had another elderly gentleman in the UK who came to me for lower back and neck pain. When I saw his posture I was not surprised he was complaining of pain in these areas. He had a poking chin and his back was totally flat just so that his head could still maintain a semi upright position. After I had assessed him and massaged his back and stuck needles in, I gave him the puppy dog lie position exercise.

Here you lie on your stomach up on your elbows forming a triangle with your hands and thumbs. You visualize you have an apple under your chin to keep your head in a good position. (You can place your fist under your chin to get the correct position and then put it back in the triangle). You then push upwards through the shoulders. Almost like doing a push up but with the arms bent. Your pelvis must stay flat on the floor. If you are very stiff you will struggle to keep the pelvis flat on the floor as it will lift off naturally. As you improve so too will your flexibility and you will be able to keep the pelvis on the floor. This strengthens the shoulder girdle and the back of your neck and stretches the anterior part of your hips. All in all this corrects your posture, getting your head back and your lower back into a better curve.

This man was diligent as usual with his exercises and within two weeks when he came for his next treatment, I did not even recognize him. When he walked in I asked if I could help him as he was this upright gentleman and not the old hunchback I saw the previous time. He laughed at me and told me he was here to see me, at which point my jaw dropped open and I asked him what he had been doing that had made him look so fabulous. He told me he did his exercise (puppy dog lie) every day every two hours and he was feeling great. His back pain was gone and so was his neck pain. So too was the awful posture. Working with the British made me realize the importance of exercise and doing it regularly.

Joe Pilates states that within 10 sessions, you feel a difference, within 20 sessions you see a difference and within 30 sessions you have a new posture. This is truly what I have experienced in my practice.

It does not matter which exercise you like to do, as long as you do it. If you do have a specific problem however, you need to focus on getting that specific muscle back into working properly and then your problems should go away. You also need to ensure you have full range of movement for each area of the body as if you do not then no matter how hard you train you will not be able to do everything that you want to do. This was clear with the pole dancing lady I mentioned earlier in the book.

I am treating an elderly lady who has been struggling to lift up her arm for almost a year. She has been scared to come for physio. When I first saw her she was unable to lift her arm when lying on her back as it would click and groan and be too painful. After 2 weeks, she was able to lift the arm lying on her back and after another week was able to lift the arm in standing. Many of you may be asking why she could lift the arm while lying on her back but not in standing. This is due to gravity playing resistance on the arm. When you stand, you have to lift your arm against gravity, but when you are lying down, gravity actually helps the arm a bit. I always start training the arm muscles while the patient is lying on their back or their side. A bent arm is also easier to start with. You can even use the good arm to help lift it, if both your arms are useless, then you get someone to help you lift it, or you make a pulley and use that to help you lift the arm up.

We use a grading scale to determine how weak your body is. They call it the Oxford grading scale.

Grade 1 is a flicker, Grade 2 is when you are able to lift the arm in supine without gravity, grade 3 is when you can lift the arm while standing, grade 4 is when you can lift your arm with a light weight while standing, grade 5 is excellent strength and you are able to lift heavy weights while standing. You can vary the grades by having a grade 2- or grade 2+, which is when you can either just not lift the arm without gravity, or you can lift the arm without gravity with a weight, but are just not able to lift the arm in standing without a weight. So the lady I mentioned above, had Grade 2- strength when I first saw her, she now has a grade 3-. This is when she is just able to lift the arm in standing, but needs a little bit of help. She is quite easily able to do a grade 2+, so we are almost there. By improving her strength in her arms, she has reduced her pain significantly and has also reduced the grinding and groaning the shoulder was making. Weakness is a terrible thing and many people think that because they are walking fine and doing their normal daily living things, even sport that they are fine and that they are not weak.

What do I mean by this? I was treating a young man. He was complaining of lower back pain for many years and he does rock climbing and martial arts as his recreational sport. When I first evaluated him I did a quick buttock strength test which indicated that his gluteus medius was weak as he was unable to stand on one leg while I was applying resistance to the same side over his hip area. This meant to me that his buttock was weak and could be the cause of his back pain. Gluteus medius refers pain to the lower back area. It is also the muscle that is partly responsible for you standing in an upright posture. He had a flattened back and was very stiff with bending forward. I started to release the buttocks and hamstrings and gave him a buttock strengthening exercise.

Within a week he reported that his back pain was significantly better. When I told this to one of my older patients, who had been loath to do the exercises, he promptly started exercising that day and also within a week reported being much improved. Unfortunately when you stop exercising you may lose the strength and may experience the same pain at a later stage. So try to continue to exercise on a regular basis to keep up your general flexibility and strength.

With all my knowledge of how to exercise and the importance of exercising, I too fell into the trap of not exercising. Firstly after my car accident when I did exercise I would experience such severe headaches, that I came to a grinding halt with my hockey and cycling and gardening. Every now and then I would attempt to cycle a short distance and regret the attempt. What one must remember is that when you have suffered an injury or you have not exercised for a very long time for whatever reason, be it pain, fatigue, or whatever, you need to start like a snail. If you have had an injury, you need to have someone help release the tight areas while you gradually increase your exercises. Exercise on its own does not always work.

I tell my patients that there is a very fine line between doing exercise right and getting improved results, or crossing over the line and bemoaning the fact that you will never get better. This is detrimental as you can go into depression and believe that you will never get better. This is why it is vital to be guided by a physiotherapist or other therapist who can help you in the beginning phases and then later with a Biokineticist who can help you with the end rehabilitation phase.

One of my patients', who has severe body pain, is so sore she is unable to lift her leg to climb onto my treatment bed. I need to drop it to its lowest point. She is also unable to sit on the floor or do any form of exercise. With the treatments, she has been steadily improving and has started walking on a treadmill. She was up to 30min on the treadmill at a slow pace, when she decided that she would increase the time and the speed. This was a huge mistake as the next day she felt sore all over and was quite despondent thinking she had regressed.

The fact was that she had crossed that fine line of doing just too much. This caused her to get muscle stiffness which is felt as pain as she is not that active yet. Since then she has gradually increased her exercise regime continuing with her physio each week. She was able to join a gym and attended 3 sessions per week with a personal trainer, some months after starting treatment. We continued to release her body and now she is able to attend 4 sessions per week with a personal trainer where before any exercise was too painful.

So how does one progress your exercises. You must first increase the time you exercise. You do this for about a week. Then you increase the speed at which you walk, but keep the time the same. This is done for a week. If you have managed to walk for that speed easily, you can then increase the time again. If you have reached the time you want to walk for, and then increase the speed steadily until you have reached the speed you wish to walk or start to jog and gradually increase the speed to running, if this is what you want to do. For this lady she has improved so much that she was able to start training 3 times a week at a gym with an instructor. She has been doing this for some months now and is feeling so good that she has added a fourth session at the gym and has also added a Pilates class and a water aerobics class. She has improved so much that she feels she is ready to find work again and as she has not found anything for 6 months has decided to offer her time up at the animal shelter to keep herself busy and not get depressed. I have been really impressed with her progress and dedication to improve her health in all aspects.

If you don't have someone to show you how to do the Pilates exercises then you can do the following. This I heard on a CD by a gentleman who used to train gymnasts. One of his students came up to him and asked the coach if there was something he could do to have a better looking body and get his muscles to have definition. The coach asked what he was currently doing, was he at the gym, swimming, what? To which the student replied that he was doing nothing. The coach then suggested that he do 10 push-ups, 10 squats, 10 sit-ups and 10 back exercises. The athlete looked at him and told him that that was ridiculous as it was nothing. To which the coach replied "It is not nothing, it is 10 push-ups, 10 sit-ups, 10 squats and 10 back exercises." The student looked at him as if he was mad, but agreed to do the exercises daily.

6 Months down the line the athlete was approached by some team mates and asked what he was doing to look so trim and good. The athlete answered that he had been doing 10 sit-ups, 10 squats, 10 push-ups and 10 back exercises. They looked at him and laughed saying that it was nothing, at which point he said "It's not nothing, its 10 push-ups, 10 squats, 10 sit-ups and 10 back exercises."

I broke it down into 10 squats, 10 wall push ups, 10 Pilates sit-ups, and 10 bridging exercises. Of course if you can't do these exercises, then you modify the modified Pilates exercises and do what you can do, but just get moving and get stronger. I had one of my elderly gentlemen do the above regime and he was pleased to inform me recently that he has started getting definition in his thighs. So even at his age he can also cut muscles and look good.

In a short period of time you will reap the benefits. If you are unable to motivate yourself, make sure you rope in the little police men in the form of grandkids or kids as they are only too willing to do them with you. If you are not fortunate to have any of them, then get your spouse and if you still don't have one of them, then show your cat or dog what you can do. I am sure they will watch you and think you are doing either something funny and get excited or think you are daft. Either way it will amuse them. My dog Paddington even joins us for a few of the exercises. He thinks he's a little human boy.

I had a young girl who had just turned 16 so was referred to the adult department in the UK for treatment. She was complaining of severe right knee pain and the surgeons had looked at her X-rays and decided that if physio did not work, then they would have to operate and break her leg and turn it 8 degrees as her leg was not in alignment. This leg pain had been there for a few months and when I asked what she had been doing when the leg started hurting she told me that she had never done exercises before and then signed up to do the paper run. This meant that she had to get up early in the morning and cycle for 2 hours each day to drop off all the papers. I knew immediately that she had overworked her legs as they had never done exercise prior to this paper run and that they were complaining profusely.

When I palpated her legs I could feel the muscle spasms all over the thighs like speed bumps down the legs. I inserted the needles and massaged her legs and within 4 sessions her pain was gone. As her legs were very weak generally, I recommended the Pilates exercises attached at the end of the chapter. She did these exercises religiously as they all do and even converted their garage into a gym. Most of the folks in the UK ride the bus and don't have cars. She was feeling fine and was discharged from my care. It must have been about 6 months later when she decided to come visit me and show me how well she was doing. It is always nice to hear from my patients out of the blue like this.

She came into the department and I just remember those amazing She-Ra legs. They had gone from the ugly duckling thin sticks to really nice defined muscular legs. She enjoyed exercising so much that she had added more gym equipment and was training her whole body. It was so nice to see.

I had another young girl also about the same age as the previous story. She however, did not have any injury, but due to her weak muscles would have her knee caps dislocate regularly. She was complaining of pain in both her knees and was unable to sit to watch any long movies as her knees would become unbearably painful and she would be unable to straighten them. If they were straight then she would be unable to bend them. They were uncomfortable when she slept and the Doctors where thinking of doing a lateral knee release if Physio didn't work. Here they cut the little muscle on the outside of the knee to prevent it from pulling the knee cap outwards and dislocating it.

I started with the needles again and the massage, but the most important aspect of the treatment was the Pilates exercises. She too did them religiously and she had improved leg strength and definition. Her legs were too weak to maintain balance of the patella which is why it dislocated. By improving the strength in her legs, she no longer had dislocation of her patella and she no longer had knee pain as she had full range of movement and she did not need to go for surgery.

Although these people have all done the exercises and recovered, it was a long recovery for some of them. Some of them needed to have treatment first to loosen the muscles so that they could do the movement before they could do the exercises. Some of my patients need to be motivated for a long time before they even consider doing the exercises, but each of them is a process that needs to be gone through. Some unfortunately never get round to exercising and then live in pain.

I had a young man whose shoulders dislocated all the time. Even when he lifted his arms they would dislocate and they would dislocate at about 20 degrees of lifting, it was very bad. Once again we had to start doing exercises and he had to do them regularly and he was not allowed to let his shoulders dislocate when he did his exercises. So we had a very small range of movement in which to work. He was not allowed to use it as a party trick and he was no allowed to do any contact sport for a year. He used to play rugby and squash. We started the long haul with modified Pilates' exercises and bingo wings. A bingo wing is an exercise I created using a ruler. You literally flap the ruler back and forth while your arm fixed so that it only works in the shoulder. This helps activate the ligaments and small muscles around the shoulder which pulls the shoulder back into the socket.

He had to do this exercise every two hours and was not allowed to let the shoulder feel unsafe or dislocate. Once again it took us 6 months of regular exercising and gradually increasing his exercises. When he could reach 90 degrees without his shoulder dislocating, he joined our shoulder rehabilitation class and was not allowed to go above 90 degrees. At the end of his treatment we were doing bingo wing with his arm at the top in a tennis serve position. He was told he could return to his sport as his shoulder no longer dislocated and he had good muscle control and strength.

I have gone through many different techniques in this book and sometimes we need to do all of them before we reach the exercises. Remember exercise is number 5 on the 6 fundamental factors and thus sometimes it is also no 5 in the queue of things to do. So don't beat yourself up about not exercising when you are not able to anyway. When the time is right you will want to exercise and then you can get someone to help you get going.

When I finally got my energy back and was ready to exercise I thought I would start by walking around the block. To my horrors I was stiff the next morning in my legs. I know that because of my adrenal fatigue and the fact that I had no energy to do any exercises that I would be weak but I did not expect it to be this bad. What actually made me realize that it was that bad was when I went for a Body composition Analysis.

How this body composition analysis works, is you stand on a very smart machine that looks like a scale, but you also hold electrodes in your hand. You then watch a monitor in front of you that shows you how it scans the right leg then left leg, the right arm and left arm and then your body. It was very interesting to watch and even more interesting to get the results. I knew I was struggling a bit with a little tummy and that I was not fighting fit, but because my work is physical and I am always standing and massaging I thought my arms were strong and my legs were strong. Also I have been dancing for 4 years and although it's not intense it is a little workout and this is done once a week.

When I read my analysis I decided that I have kiewiet syndrome. My arms and legs are literally just sticks with hardly any muscle mass and I have a fat stomach of 34% body fat, but yet my BMI is normal. Basically my muscles have disappeared from the lack of exercise due to the fatigue. It's strange though because I have strong arms and can lift heavy objects and have definition of my triceps and biceps so you would think the muscle mass was good.

With many of my patients I have noticed that when you are in pain or when you have fatigue, you have a tendency to not exercise as it causes more pain or more fatigue. So we avoid doing what we know is good for us, because at that time it really is not good for us. Luckily one can resolve the issues by ensuring you fix the imbalance of your minerals in your body and when your energy levels are back to normal you can start working on the Kiewiet syndrome.

I remember when I was newly qualified, I decided to put a hockey team together who would play against the university teams. It was a social team and we never practiced together, we only pitched for the game and then warmed our jaws up chatting and went onto the field to play. The games were only 10minutes a side but this is very long, when you are not fit. So I would change into my hockey gear while driving to the game and play the 20minutes.

This one evening the physio university team was a man short for the game after ours, so I gladly volunteered to play as well. I remember during the game how my hamstrings, calves and quads all cramped at the same time. I told the goalie to get out the box and go play and I would defend the box, because I could no longer run. This was the Thursday night and the next morning I was a bit stiff, but as all of you know it's the second day after that which is the worst and I was working the weekend.

I remember having to drive to 5 different hospitals and taking so long to get out the car as every muscle in my body was screaming with pain. I do not know how I managed to get through the day, but I started at 6 am and finished at 6pm and then came down with a cold to top it all off. Worst of all was that I had to repeat it all over again on the Sunday. I had definitely overdone it even though it was fun. Don't take it to the extreme as you will also cry and curse yourself for days afterwards.

There is also a fine line when you must start exercising to get improvement. This brings me to another few stories. I had this British man who had injured his left shoulder falling off his horse and we had been working on it for months increasing range of movement and his pain was bearable but was not gone. He was also scared to go riding again as his arm was too painful and he was scared he would cause more damage. In the end I told him that he needs to get back to his riding as we have hit a brick wall and we are not getting improvement there because there is weakness and the only way to fix the weakness is to go and exercise. So he went and when he returned the week after he reported that his shoulder pain had gone.

The other thing you can do to combat Kiewiet syndrome is to walk around the block. This I do while mostly talking to every neighbour I come across, but still walking and getting out there. I walk with my son and we get time to chat about school and things going on in his life. You are getting out absorbing Vitamin D which is essential in your body functioning properly. 85% of South Africans are Vitamin D deficient. Make sure you are not one of them. Walking is not going to fix Kiewiet syndrome, because your weak muscle will still stay weak. Your buttock muscle will not strengthen by walking around the block, they will improve but you learn to cheat by using the stronger muscles when walking and doing your daily routine, so you need to do both. This boils down to doing cardio, which is the walking around the block and core, which is the 4 x 10 exercises of bridge, Pilates sit-ups, wall push-ups and squats. Slow and easy does it with exercise. There are good You Tube videos with various exercises and durations that will help provide variety and a simple routine.

It has been shown that more than 1 hour of TV for a young child will decrease their gross motor development and they will have poor posture and resultant pain in the form of back or neck pain and headaches. Many of our children have poor postures, with slouching shoulders and poking chins with a flat back. It is caused from sitting either in front of the TV, iPad or reading for long periods of time with a poor posture. To compensate for this, it is vital to work on good posture. This is done through focusing on the Pilates posture recommended and using this posture when doing your exercises. Make sure you exercise 3-4 times per week or more and cut back on your time using these devices if possible and make sure that when you are working on these devices that your ergonomics is correct.

EARLY STABILISATION EXERCISES

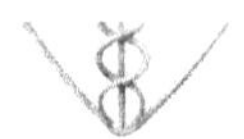

SETTING / CENTERING:

FIND NEUTRAL SPINE - Flatten small of back down into bed and then arch away from bed. Neutral spine is the middle of these two movements. (Where pubic bone and hip bone level).

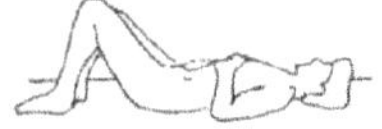

SET DEEP ABDOMINALS - Maintain neutral spine. Relax shoulders and breathing. As you breathe out gently set deep abdominals by either:

1. Gently squeeze and lift pelvic floor, as if stopping yourself passing water. Or…
2. Gently pull in abdomen below your tummy button.

Feel a gentle tension across your lower abdomen. Hold this tension and breathe normally for 10 cycles. Repeat minimum 3 times daily,
Repeat above action when sitting, standing, walking and with activity.

HIP TWIST:

Lying on your back with both knees bent. Find your neutral spine.
Gently set your deep abdominals.

Maintain the above. Exhale to start and slowly roll one knee to the side (aim for 45°)
Inhale and return knee to start position.

Repeat________times left and right, ________ times a day.

LEG STRETCH:

Lying on your back with both knees bent. Find neutral spine.
Gently set your deep abdominals.

Maintain the above. Exhale to start and stretch leg out (keep foot on floor). Inhale and return to start position. (Alternate left to right to challenge control).

Repeat ______ times left and right.__________times a day.

SHOULDER BRIDGE:

Lying on your back with both knees bent. Find neutral spine.
Gently set your deep abdominals.

Squeeze your bottom muscles. Exhale and roll your pelvis back and peal your spine off the floor, vertebra by vertebra. Inhale to hold and exhale to lower to starting position.

Repeat __________ times,______________ times a day.

DOUBLE ARM LIFT:

Lying on your back with both knees bent and arms at your side. Find neutral spine.
Gently set your deep abdominals.

Maintain the above. Exhale and raise arms up and over your head (keep ribs to the floor). Inhale and return to start position.

Repeat__________ times,____________ times a day

CLAM:

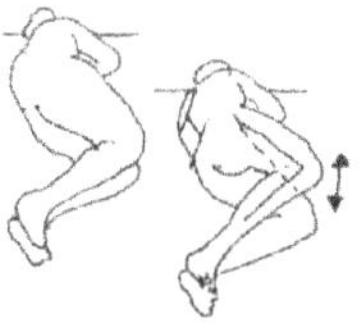

Lie on your side with both knees bent, ankles stacked on top ofeach other.
Gently set your deep abdominals. Squeeze bottom muscles.

Maintain the above. Exhale to start and float the top knee up (keeping feet together on bed). Inhale and slowly lower. DO NOT LET TRUNK ROLE FORWARD OR BACK...!

Repeat__________times, left and right__________times a day.

PRONE KNEE BEND:

Lying on your stomach, legs stretched behind.
Gently set your deep abdominals. Squeeze bottom muscles

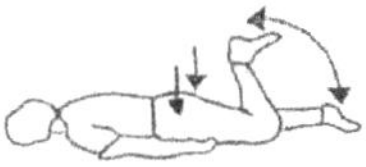

Maintain the above. Exhale to start and one bend knee. Inhale to return to start position. Alternate left and right.

Repeat__________times, left and right__________times a day.

SCAPULA SETTING:

Lying on your stomach, head supported on pillow arms at your side.
Gently set your deep abdominals.

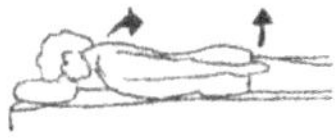

Squeeze bottom muscles, set shoulders square (down and back). Exhale to start and float arms up from floor. Inhale to lower. Relax bottom and shoulders.

Repeat__________times,__________times a day.

KNEELING ARM LIFT:

On your hands and knees. Spine positioned in neutral.
Gently set your deep abdominals.

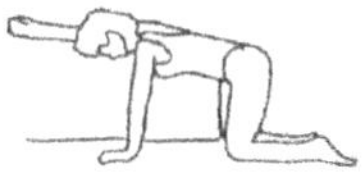

Maintain the above. Exhale to start and float arm forward and up. Inhale to lower. (Alternate left to right to challenge control).

Repeat__________times, left and right__________times a day.

STANDING HEEL LIFT:

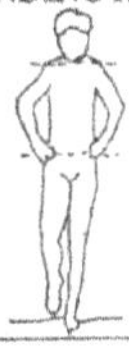

Standing, knees soft, spine positioned in neutral hands on hips.
Gently set deep abdominals.

Exhale to start and slowly lift heel from floor (progress to lifting entire foot).
MAINTAIN LEVEL PELVIS WITH MINIMAL SWAY...!

Repeat__________times, left and right__________times a day.

FUNCTIONAL INTEGRATION:

Try to maintain a neutral posture and set deep abdominal muscles during everyday functional activities. Eg. Washing up, Ironing, Lifting, walking the dog, making the bed, sitting on the bus, brushing teeth, putting on shoes and socks....!

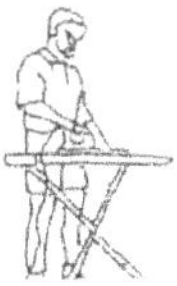

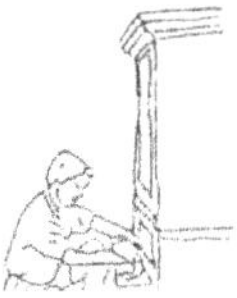

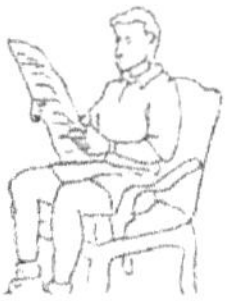

Chapter 15
Sleep

The last fundamental factor of being healthy is sleep. I think people underestimate how important sleep is. I was attending a seminar and on the seminar the lecturer was telling us a story about this gentleman who was born in Australia and when he was an adult had moved to the USA. A few years after his move he became very ill and no Doctor could tell him what the problem was and nothing he did changed his symptoms. He finally came to this lecturers' door and they were going through the lifestyle changes of the 6 fundamental factors when it was clearly shown that the time zone difference had influenced his health. He had changed everything else expect this factor; he flew home to test the theory. His symptoms went away and he had to make the decision of whether he was prepared to stay in America or move back to Australia.

During the day your body releases a hormone called cortisol. This hormone peaks at 8am and plateaus during the day until it is exchanged with melatonin at night to help you sleep properly. Cortisol is important for driving the body during the day. It is the chemical that gives us the energy to get through the day.

If you do not have enough cortisol then you will feel tired during the day, you will have trouble concentrating and you will find things more stressful than they should be. You can also have your cortisol spiking at the wrong time if you are changing your sleep patterns around which can cause a big problem. Probably what happened with the man in the USA?

Melatonin is important for having a good nights' sleep and ensures that you are well rested the next day. If you do not go to bed in time, then your cortisol will still be released, as it is released with any light that shines on the body. Thus if you do go to bed and you have a bed side light on, this will keep your cortisol levels elevated. If you have a digital watch in the room or the street lights are shining through the curtains, all these lights will cause your body to continue to release cortisol, which will firstly continue to deplete the stores and secondly prevent melatonin from taking over and doing its job.

In one of the episodes of Fifth Gear they actually did a little test on this and had a small light shine on their body during an airplane flight and measured the cortisol release in the body, indicating that even a red point finder light through a blanket was enough to activate the cortisol. This means that you need to ensure that you have no lights or electronic equipment like TVs in your room. You can get block out material that you sew onto the back of your curtains to prevent the street lights shining through the curtains at night. Most of the hotels have this, which is why you are disorientated when you wake up and it is still so dark and you are certain that it is still the middle of the night, when in fact it is time to get up or much later thank you think!

On the course we also learnt that one should be going to bed about 2 hours after sunset. So for us in South Africa it means about 9pm in the summer and about 7h30pm in the winter. I am sure that most of you have found that in the winter when it is about 7h30pm, that you feel as though it is later and you need to be asleep. Instead you stay up because you feel guilty going to bed at that hour of the day and make sure you wait till at least 9pm or later when you think it is a better time to go to bed.

Many people just stay up late because they have work to do or watch too much TV. I have found that when I get a new series that I really enjoy I am able to watch quite a few without feeling tired. I then land up staying up late for about 2 weeks in a row as you get enthralled in the story. The problem with this is that after the two weeks, I am tired and grumpy and don't feel like working and when I get exposed to germs I will definitely get sick as my immune system has been compromised from lack of sleep. Your immune system is not the only thing that is compromised from lack of sleep. It has been shown that lack of sleep can cause weight gain and diabetes as your insulin is also still active because you are up late. All your systems are compromised.

I have noticed when my son does not get to bed early it affects him for two days. He cries more and throws tantrums and is unpleasant to be around. When he was little I was very specific about his sleep routines as this is vital for babies. I would clock watch and make sure that when he did make a little noise that I would pop him into bed before he was overtired and cried or was past the tired phase and turned into zombie phase. He would wake early in the morning and before he could even walk I would tell him "it is still dark outside, so not time to get up yet." I would give him some milk and he would nod off to sleep again until 8am. He would then be awake for a few hours where he would eat and play and when I saw him rub his eyes, I knew he was tired and it was time for a nap again.

Many children do not want to sleep due to excitement happening around them, or they may be worried that you will go when they go to sleep. I would always tell him that I was going to be busy at home with my work and when he wakes up we will all still be here. If I needed to go, I would tell him that I was going to pop out, but that he would be looked after by, and I would give him the persons' name. I would tell him what time I would be back in his language, by telling him that I would be back after his nap or when he was eating his lunch.

As he got to about 2 years old and he would rub his eyes and do a little moan. I would tell him: "You are crying because you are tired, or hungry," or whichever one it was according to the time. "Go and climb in your bed and have a nap, I am not going anywhere, see you when you wake up." Or if he was hungry "go and look in the fridge for an apple and some nuts, bring them here and eat them while I am busy here with this patient." He would crawl to the kitchen open the fridge and bring the items and sit and eat them while I was busy.

When he was about 2 and a half, he came to me the one day and told me that he was tired and asked if it was okay to go and lie down. He really understood what the different feelings were and was able to help himself just because he had the knowledge. Now when he stays up late and he is grumpy the next day, I point it out to him and explain why he is feeling the way he is feeling. This will be very powerful knowledge in his future as he will know how to avoid it and what it is if he does do it on a regular basis.

Just before he turned three I stopped my sons' day naps. The reason for this was that he was staying up later at night after a nap because he was not tired and then he didn't want to wake up in the morning because he had gone to bed too late. So we stopped the napping, but I made sure he went to bed a little earlier. His bed time at this age was about 4h30pm-5pm, once down he would be lights out within 5 minutes and he would sleep till the next morning 5am or even later at 6h30am, sleeping on average for about 13 hours. As he got older his bed time would gradually get later but only by about 30min each year. He was still going to bed at 5pm when he was 5 and 5h30 when he was 6 and 6pm when he was seven. This time has been there till he was 8 when he went to bed at 7pm and now at the age of 10 he is able to go to bed at 7h30pm with sometimes going to bed at 8pm. Some days however, I can see he is tired and then chase him to bed a little earlier. But on the weekends I know he is tired because he sleeps till 7am-8am, which is still early but one should be waking up with the sun.

If you need an alarm clock to wake up, then you are not getting enough sleep.

Time	High	Low
11am-1pm	Heart	Gall Bladder
1pm-3pm	Small intestine	Liver
3pm-5pm	Bladder	Lung
5pm-7pm	Kidney	Large Intestine
7pm-9pm	Pericardium	Stomach
9pm-11pm	Triple Heater (San Jiao)	Spleen
11pm-1am	Gall Bladder	Heart
1am-3am	Liver	Small Intestine
3am-5am	Lung	Bladder
5am-7am	Large Intestine	Kidney
7am-9am	Stomach	Pericardium
9am-11am	Spleen	Triple Heater

Your body has a certain time that it does housecleaning for each of the organs. If you are not asleep during that specific time when that organ gets its house cleaning done, then it misses out on it and you get a back log of toxins in that organ and can have problems linked with that organ.

Perhaps if you find that you are constantly waking between 1-3am one should consider doing a liver cleanse to help this organ detox properly. Similarly for 3-5am when your lungs are working hard, one can do a lung cleanse too. When you are unhealthy it is always wise to start with the intestines first as this is where it all starts.

When you eat your food, you need to digest it properly and be able to eliminate on a daily basis. If you are not eliminating waste on a daily basis you need to ensure you get this working pronto. Once this is working you can consider doing a liver cleanse.

Ensure you do not have any gall stones and if you do have gall stones that they are not too large to pass. The liver cleanse will get your gall bladder to strongly contract and you can actually eliminate little gall stones without having to remove your gall bladder.

Once this has been done you can look into repairing the gut lining to ensure you do not have leaky gut. Leaky gut is seen through bloating, indigestion, diarrhoea, constipation, nutrient malabsorption, fatigue, multiple food sensitivities, allergies and intolerances, skin allergy, lowered immunity, depression, brain fog, skin rashes, memory loss, ADHD, seasonal allergies or asthma, hormonal imbalances such as PMS or PCOS, autoimmune disease such as rheumatoid arthritis, Hashimoto's, lupus, psoriasis or celiac disease. This is a large range of diseases and more information can be found on this through the Functional medicine institute.

I remember treating a five year old child who was still having two naps in the day, one early morning at about 10am and then another one at about 4pm. This meant that he was up until 11pm or even 12pm as he was not tired enough to go to bed. So his parents would have to stay up with him and they were totally exhausted. I advised that they cut out his day naps altogether and focus on getting him to bed early in the night. This would mean that they would have some time to relax before having to go to bed. Whether they did it or not, I don't know. She had no idea that this was the cause of the problems.

Recently I was treating another lady and we started talking about sleep and the importance of it, when she mentioned that her son who is now 4 also has a day nap and then only wants to go to bed late at night, I advised this sleeping pattern to her. She has implemented it and reports that it is going very well and that she is able to get to bed earlier herself which has helped for her mental state and fatigue in her own body.

Below is the Epworth Sleeping scale. This you can complete to see how effectively you are sleeping. There are several medical problems that can influence sleep, but avoid sleeping in the day as this will prevent you from sleeping properly at night. The only time you can sleep in the day is when you are sick with the Flu and need to be in bed, or if you are trying to recover from adrenal fatigue. If you are tired you may go to bed earlier but you should wake before the alarm clock the next day. Really listen to your body and do what it is telling you to do.

Epworth Sleeping scale

- **0- No chance of dozing**
- **1- Slight chance of dozing**
- **2 – moderate chance of dozing**
- **3- high chance of dozing**

- Sitting reading
- Watching TV
- Sitting inactive in public place (theatre)
- As passenger in car without a break for 1hr
- Lying down for rest in afternoon when permitted.
- Sitting talking to someone
- Sitting quietly after lunch without alcohol
- In a car when stopped for a few minutes in traffic

Score

- 1-6 getting enough sleep
- 7-8 Score is average
- 9+ Seek the advice of a sleep specialist

There are many things that you can do to improve your sleep. Sometimes it is as simple as getting into a routine as you would do for a child. Make sure your routine stays the same. Perhaps you could do with some relaxation as you may have had a busy day and are exhausted, but find it hard to switch off the mind. In cases like this you may find it beneficial to have a relaxing bath/shower before you go to bed.

Try keeping your bed time the same time every night. If you are going to bed very late, after 10h30pm because you are unable to sleep, then try using a routine to calm you down and slowly bring your sleeping time earlier by 15 minutes every week until you reach the desired time of 10-10h30pm every night at the latest.

If you are unable to switch the mind off, then try reading a boring book that is guaranteed to make you drowsy. You could also listen to classical music that lulls you to sleep. My son listens to a story every night; this could also work for you. Make sure that you cover the light of the CD player so that it does not disturb your sleep. I use a mini Persian carpet draped over the radio so the light is not seen.

There is also a technique you can use, similar to counting sheep. You must continue with this technique until it works for you. If you stop before your body has become used to the routine, then this technique will not work for you. What you do is close your eyes while lying in bed. Visualize that you are drawing an X in your mind and then draw a circle surrounding the X. Then imagine yourself taking a cloth and rub it out and replace it with 100, keeping the circle in place. Repeat this counting backwards 99-98-97-96......, each time rubbing the number out before writing the next one. Personally I do not get very far as I get confused as to which number I had before this one and then before I know it I have drifted off into sleep.

Often when I am struggling to fall asleep, it is because I am hungry. You may not realize that you are hungry, but if you try eat a protein snack, you may find that you drift off to sleep more easily afterwards. Make sure that it is more a protein snack than a vegetable, or fruit. Avoid drinking coffee after 3pm in the afternoon if you struggle to sleep and avoid eating chocolates and drinking anything with caffeine in it. One must also avoid drinking too much water after 3pm in the afternoon as you will wake up regularly to urinate. You must try drinking your quota of water that you need earlier in the day. Many of my patients have mentioned before that they have water next to their beds because they get very thirsty at night. You need to retrain your body to drink in the day. You should be fast asleep at night and not wake to drink or eat. If you wake in the morning and have water next to your bed, try and drink about a glass full. This will activate your thirst reflex and I find that I tend to drink more water in the day then and am able to finish my quota of water before 3 pm in the afternoon. I am still able to drink a bit after 3pm, but it's not as much as if I don't drink during the day and then I sleep much better and don't have to get up during the night.

With the adrenal fatigue I had, nothing I did worked and I would lie for hours waiting to fall asleep. During this period I tried taking some Melatonin tablets, which is what your body would normally release during the night. This helped me and has helped some of my other patients who have similar problems and also suffer from the adrenal fatigue. Each person is different and not everything will work the same way for everyone, so be prepared to try different things until you find the one that works for you.

Other patients are overweight and then have sleep apnea which means you stop breathing and then snore yourself awake. For this you need to firstly eat more healthily as mentioned earlier. Lose some of the weight so that your throat doesn't close from the weight. Try getting used to sleeping on your side instead of your back, again so you do not close your airway. A C-PAP machine is often recommended. This machine forces air into your chest at regular intervals and prevents you from taking shallow breaths.

Perhaps your Vit D is low and your calcium and magnesium are low which can cause cramping at night waking you. Or perhaps you are in pain and need to find someone to help ease the pain so that you can sleep properly. We have discussed many components in this book and hopefully you will find the ones that will work for you. If you are taking Vitamin D, please ensure you measure your levels regularly as it is a fat soluble vitamin and gets stored in your fat and can result in you getting too much Vit D.

One of my patients was telling me that she was struggling to sleep. Recently it came out that she was unable to sleep at night, because she was having a little day nap because she would lie in front of the TV as there was nothing else to do and then go to sleep. We had a discussion in one of our sessions where we were talking about getting busy and doing more around the house. She has not been able to get a job for the past 6 months due to specific regulations in our country and was feeling depressed. I suggested that if she wants more she needs to do more. This means, if you can't get a job, don't sit at home and bemoan the fact that you don't have work, get out there and get busy. Perhaps you can work in your garden, or do cooking for the freezer for when you do get a job and don't have time to cook. She did not have freezer space so when she came to the next session, she told me that she had decided to do more exercises and joined another 2 exercise groups, which meant she went from walking only about 4000 steps per day to about 11 000 steps per day. Since she was so much more active she was physically tired at the end of the day and thus popped right off to sleep.

She has decided to study further to ensure she becomes more diverse to have more options for work and to add to her hire-ability and she decided to volunteer her time at our SPCA to help the people there deal with their difficult situations as this is what she is trained to do. So she is making a plan to become busy and keep active and feel like she is needed in society. This has significantly improved her mental wellbeing and she feels much improved physically and is sleeping better.

If you are not sure how your quality of sleep is, it may be worth getting something that can measure it. I have a fit bit which measures the quality and quantity of sleep I have as well as my steps and the amount of water I drink for the day. You can even add what you have eaten. This gets charted, enabling you to monitor your progress over a period of time. I found it useful when determining how Vincent was sleeping.

If I get my 10 000 steps in for the day, I sleep soundly and wake rested the next morning. If I only get 8000 steps in, then I am often restless through the night. Drinking enough fluid before 3pm in the afternoon, with small amounts thereafter and walking the 10 000 steps for the day makes me sleep wonderfully. Perhaps getting a simple tool like this can help keep you motivated to do all the right things.

Conclusion

I have shared a lot of information in this book with you and many of my patients have been begging me to write it for a long time now. There were a few things that pushed me forward to reaching the point where I decided it was now or never in writing this book. One of them was the dog bite that I had two years prior to writing this book.

I was wondering what all these incidents in my life were telling me to do after the bite, and perhaps this book is that answer. There is a lot of information and answers one can share when you experience life in all its different aspects. Perhaps your journey you are going through will also lead you to write a book which will help many people overcome similar problems. Your way of looking at life is different to mine and you will have learnt different things and the way you write will speak to different people than the way I write.

Second aspect that guided me to write this book was reading all the self-empowerment books that come to me in the post. I realized that most of the people were writing as if they were talking to me and their thoughts were often seen as common knowledge and made a lot of sense to me. Sometimes what they wrote was what I had felt in my gut but had not been able to express in words. I realized that their writing was for the everyday person who is looking for answers and it's just their thoughts they are putting to pen and paper that has helped millions of people across the world. As my English was never seen as great at school I never thought I was good enough to write a book, but having people proof read your books and correct your spelling and grammar enables you to get the information across in a readable format.

Thirdly I had a patient with chronic pain who had seen many of the top Physios in South Africa and he looked me up on the internet and decided to come and see me. These top Physios have also written books and are seen as icons in our industry. When he told me that he thought I was really good, it empowered me to share my knowledge in this book format.

Of course I would not be able to test all my new found knowledge I have gained through all my experiences and courses if I did not have my patients who were all willing guinea pigs to try anything that I was willing to do with them. It has been a joy treating them, as they are all eager to do what I ask. Hearing each of their stories inspires me to help them more and the more they do what I ask them to do, the more I think of for them to do. I absolutely love what I do and cannot think of anything else I would rather be doing.

I truly hope that this information in this book has guided you and motivated you to find your team to help you move forward on your path to recovery. If you do not have a team yet, then I hope this book has again motivated you to start your journey on your own.

When the student is ready, the Master appears

www.ingramcontent.com/pod-product-compliance
Ingram Content Group UK Ltd.
Pitfield, Milton Keynes, MK11 3LW, UK
UKHW021036270726
13967UKWH00013B/2808

9 780620 758642